COPING WITH THYROID PROBLEMS

DR JOAN GOMEZ is Honorary Consulting Psychiatrist to the Chelsea and Westminster Hospital. She was trained at King's College, London, and Westminster Hospital and obtained her DPM and MRCPsych in 1973 and 1974 respectively, and her Fellowship of the Royal College of Psychiatrists in 1982. She is a member of the Society for Psychosomatic Research, and the Medico-Legal Society, and a Fellow of the Royal Society of Medicine. She has been engaged in clinical work and research on the interface between psychiatry and physical medicine. Her husband was a general practitioner and they have ten children.

D0532659

Overcoming Common Problems Series

For a full list of titles please contact
Sheldon Press, Marylebone Road, London NW1 4DU

Overcoming Common Problems

COPING WITH
THYROID PROBLEMS

Dr Joan Gomez

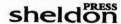
sheldon**PRESS**

First published in Great Britain 1994
Sheldon Press, SPCK, Marylebone Road, London NW1 4DU

© Dr Joan Gomez 1994

Third impression 1997

British Library Cataloguing-in-Publication Data

A catalogue record for this book is available from the British Library

ISBN 0–85969–687–1

Photoset by Deltatype Ltd, Ellesmere Port, Cheshire
Printed and bound in Great Britain by
Biddles Ltd, Guildford and King's Lynn

Contents

Introduction

I have a fellow feeling for people with thyroid problems because they have cropped up in my family too. The very first thing I did when I became a doctor was to take my mother along to a thyroid specialist. My mother had an unsightly bulge in the front of her neck – easily cured, although she'd had it as long as I could remember. Much later there was my daughter, a brilliant student who started slowing down, not coping. But by that time I had developed my interest in the thyroid and the problem was nipped in the bud.

It may have been quite a shock to you when your doctor suggested doing thyroid tests. Perhaps you had gone to see him in the hope of a tonic, something to buck you up because you were feeling so down – tired, sluggish, cold all the time and, to add to your discomfort, constipated. Everything seemed to take twice as long and twice the effort, and all this had all crept up on you so sneakily. If the answer from the test came back 'underactive thyroid' you are in luck.

The treatment consists of tiny white tablets to supplement your own supply of thyroid hormone. They work like magic, and have no side-effects. You will feel yourself gradually coming back to life again – and shedding those few unwanted pounds in the process.

An underactive thyroid is a common disorder, and it can affect you at any age, but it is rather more likely as you get older. On the other hand you may have wanted help with something quite different – your nerves. You may have started feeling anxious all the time, for no reason. You can't sit still, you fly off the handle at the slightest thing, and your heart keeps thumping. Although your appetite is enormous, you are losing weight, and that is a worry. Sometimes such symptoms seem to come on after a shock, but usually no one knows why, out of the blue, the thyroid gland has started overworking.

Fortunately there is a range of medicines that will calm it down, and your mind and your heart will follow suit. Your body will run at its normal, peaceful pace again.

It may, however, be your child you are worried about – he or she isn't growing as much as other children, or is shooting up faster than they are, and, either way, is not doing well at school. Again, the remedy is straightforward.

1

Thyroid problems affect women more often than men or children, and my impression is that those affected are usually particularly warm, sympathetic people. Sometimes a thyroid malfunction comes to light from some apparently unrelated symptom such as heavy, irregular periods, or hardly any; fertility difficulties; problems in swallowing; or, in some older people, high blood pressure and some heart conditions. These, too, will all respond to treatment that gets the thyroid into good, working order.

Swelling of the thyroid gland, prominent in the front of the neck, is not important in itself from the health point of view. In some cases, for instance during pregnancy, it can be normal and temporary. In others it is due to either an overactive or an underactive thyroid, and shrinks down as the thyroid problem is settled.

What will it mean, now that a thyroid disorder has been diagnosed? Particularly if your thyroid is overactive, when the disorder itself makes you nervous, you may be worried about what the treatment entails. Nearly always, it only amounts to swallowing tablets. Sometimes this is for a short course, but in the case of an underactive thyroid it may be indefinitely. None of the treatments works immediately, but a fortnight will see an end to the worst discomfort as a rule. After that it is mainly a matter of fine-tuning the dosage. With an overactive thyroid, different medicines may be needed at different stages of your recovery.

You may have heard of radioactive iodine as a treatment for an overactive thyroid. It sounds quite frightening, but it has been used for many years and it is so safe that it is now recommended even for children. All that is needed for a permanent cure is to take radioactive iodine tablets once, and wait. Because the very short-acting radiation is in iodine, the thyroid scoops it all up and it only affects the gland. The radioactivity only lasts a few hours, but the beneficial effect comes on gradually, over several months.

As in my case, thyroid problems, but not necessarily the same kind, often run in families. This is because they are mostly due to autoimmunity – the body making a mistake and reacting against itself. Since thyroid disorders are 90 per cent curable, don't worry if they crop up among your relatives. What is useful is that your doctor will be alert to them, even with the more out-of-the-way symptoms.

While you are preoccupied with digesting the news of a thyroid complaint, you won't be able to take in every word your doctor says, especially if he slips into medical jargon. In this book I want to share with you all the information you are ever likely to need about the thyroid, in understandable language and right up to date. I hope it will give you the confidence to ask questions and get the best out of discussions with your doctor. Most of all, I hope it will help you not to worry because you don't know what the disorder and its treatment involve.

Postscript   My mother had no further trouble with her thyroid and lived until she was ninety-five and my daughter is in sparkling form, long-term.

1

What your thyroid
does for you

What is so special about your thyroid? It could not have a more important role. It is in charge of the running of every part of your body, including how you feel emotionally. As you can imagine, if it goes wrong you are affected all over, whatever your age, sex or race. Yet it is an apparently insignificant slip of tissue, weighing less than an ounce. It fits so neatly into the space round the lower part of your voice-box – your larynx – that you wouldn't know it was there, unless you knew how to find it.

To locate your thyroid, look in a mirror and swallow. You will see your larynx move up and down at the front of your neck. Lean your head forward and feel each side of your larynx with your fingers and thumb. You can just detect a little bit of soft tissue closely attached to the sides of the larynx, making them feel less hard than the front part. This is your thyroid. (Its name dates from the seventeenth century and comes from the Greek for a shield – after the shape of a Minoan battle shield.)

The way the thyroid controls the body is by producing *hormones*. 'Hormones' comes from the Greek for stimulators, which is exactly what the thyroid hormones are. These chemical messengers boost activity all over the body. They travel round in the bloodstream. Since every single part of the body must have its nourishment supplied in the blood for survival, it follows that the hormones are also conveyed to every part.

Not every organ or tissue needs a particular hormone in the same amount all the time, so there is a system rather like leaving a note out for the milkman. The parts which require more thyroid hormones, for example, open up more receptors which latch on to these hormones. Fewer receptors are opened up when less hormone is required. Thus the right quantity is supplied to the right place at the time it is wanted.

The thyroid is small but so busy and important that it has a wonderfully generous blood supply. Five times its own weight of blood goes through the gland every minute.

Bodywork

The essential work of the body is called the metabolism, from the Greek for 'change'. This means taking in adequate amounts of food and processing it to provide energy to keep your heart, breathing and digestion going, to fuel your muscles as and when needed, and also to keep your brain running. It involves repair and replacement of tissues on a regular schedule, and the disposal of waste. Another metabolic task is the conversion of alcohol and medicines into a form in which your body can get rid of them. Imagine the chaos if every drink, every aspirin, you swallowed remained in your body unchanged.

One of the thyroid's most important jobs is to monitor and control your metabolic rate – the rate at which your body uses up its fuel reserve. If there are heavy calls on this from your muscles because you are playing tennis or doing a spring-clean, or from your digestive system because there is a big meal waiting to be dealt with, your metabolic rate accelerates. The orders for this come via the thyroid.

Incidentally, a meal which is high in protein is hard work to digest and stimulates this metabolic reaction much more than a fatty meal. Slimming diets used therefore to feature steak prominently, in the hope of inducing the metabolism to burn away unwanted flesh faster. The Russian diet, except for the wealthy, contains a lot of oil, and hardly any meat. This encourages the bulky figures we see in Red Square on television.

Basic metabolic rate

If you are doing nothing more energetic than, say, reading this book, your bodily functions will be just ticking over. Under thyroid guidance, your metabolic rate will sink to its basic minimum – the basic metabolic rate, or BMR. This is high throughout childhood, when active growth and making new tissues is going on, and similarly in pregnancy, another building period. It stays high for breast-feeding also.

Thyroid hormone is particularly involved in the manufacture of body protein, especially muscle tissue, either your own or an unborn baby's, or for milk production.

The BMR settles down in ordinary adult life and middle age, but decreases once more when you are into the contemplative phase of old age.

Where you live

If you move to a colder climate your BMR will rev up by as much as

50 per cent after a few weeks, under the direction of your thyroid. You have to burn your bodily fuel faster to produce more warmth. Such vital internal organs as the liver and kidneys cannot work properly unless they, at least, maintain a normal temperature, regardless of your hands and feet.

Those who live in the Arctic regions run at a consistently higher BMR, by 15 to 20 per cent, than those of us in London or New York, say. There is a small adjustment of metabolic rate between winter and summer even in temperate climates, and you will notice the instinct to take in bigger supplies of food in a cold snap.

There is a special tissue, brown fat, which is especially useful for producing heat. It is concentrated down the back. Babies and to a lesser extent young men have plenty of this material. The fat of the middle-aged has no such useful, warming function, but remains inert, padding out the figure.

If you live at a high altitude or are otherwise in a place where the concentration of oxygen is reduced, your thyroid increases your metabolic activity. Serious mountaineers have to acclimatize themselves before tackling the highest peaks. Exposure to long sunlit days also stimulates extra thyroid hormone production and increased metabolism, although hot weather has the opposite effect.

Eating and appetite

Another useful manoeuvre by your thyroid is the adjustment of both basic and short-term rates of metabolism in response to how much you eat, though not to your actual weight. If you persistently take in more than you and your muscles need, your thyroid will help to dispose of the surplus by having it burn up more rapidly. This automatically makes you feel warmer, whatever the temperature. You can see this mechanism in action when you next go to a restaurant. You are sure to spot one or two meat-eating trencher-men looking hot and flushed: they are burning fuel fast.

By contrast, if you are on short rations, either self-chosen because you are slimming or because the food is not available, your thyroid will eke out the supply by slowing down the metabolism. This is what happens in anorexia nervosa. A low metabolic rate makes you feel deadly cold, and if it continues for long your health suffers.

Appetite is influenced by the thyroid, which nudges it towards what your body really needs. Since you are a free agent, you can, of course, override this sensible guidance. If you have been off your food because of a cold or a tummy upset, as you recover you find yourself fancying simple, easy-to-digest, nourishing foods until you are back to normal. Often the thyroid damps down our appetite during the working week to balance up for a little indulgence at the weekend.

Unfortunately the influence of the thyroid on appetite and metabolic rate depends not on how fat or thin you are, but on whether you are taking in more than you can use – or less – particularly by comparison with what you have previously eaten. An overweight person who is trying to reduce, and eating very little, will have a slow metabolic rate, so that he or she is burning the food reserves only very slowly – the reverse of what is wanted. At the same time, to make matters worse, the appetite will be pressing for more!

You may have noticed that men in general have bigger appetites than women. This is because they have a higher BMR. Men's bodies have a higher proportion of muscle, and the thyroid responds to this automatically, as though more muscle means more exercise. Men have a brisker burning-off reaction if they overeat, or take exercise.

Another way the thyroid helps is by turning down the metabolism and reducing appetite during certain illnesses. This releases your body from the tasks of digestion, so that all its energies can go towards repair and recovery.

Looks

Not only your size is affected by the thyroid: it also has some influence over the glossiness and luxuriousness, or otherwise, of your hair; whether your skin is thick or delicate, dry or moist; and to some extent the shape of your face and hands. More important for how other people see you is your vitality – the physical and mental energy that shines through all you do. The thyroid has a role in both aspects.

Physical matters

The thyroid acts as a long-term pacemaker for heartbeat, breathing and other regular bodily functions such as bowel action and monthly periods. The timing of these may all be modified by circumstances. Your heart rate speeds up with excitement or physical exertion, your bowels move faster on a high-fibre diet, but the underlying rates and rhythms are set by the thyroid. Your heart rate and breathing soon settle back to these when you sit down after running for a bus.

Muscular efficiency, for sports or work, depends on the right amount of thyroid hormone. Too little and your muscles are stiff and slow to move; too much and you feel exhausted after achieving very little. Various rheumatic and joint problems are associated with thyroid disorder.

Nowadays we are constantly warned about the dangers of too high a level of cholesterol in the blood. It increases the risks of heart attack and stroke, especially for men. One of the tasks of thyroid hormone is to keep the cholesterol level in check – but this is a vain attempt in the seriously fat.

Emotional balance

Health is usually considered from the physical aspect, but you are not just a body. The essential you is in your mind and personality. Your get-up-and-go, your mental energy, depends on an adequate supply of thyroid hormone. If this is normal you will be alert but not on edge, and your concentration will be spot-on. You will be able to express yourself without difficulty and solve day-to-day problems, in the absence of illness or a major disaster.

More importantly, for a happy life, if your thyroid is in balance, so too will be your judgement. You will neither panic over trivia nor sink into helpless despair at the first set-back. You will steer between unrealistic optimism and the propensity to see only the black side. Sexual feeling – libido – and ordinary friendliness also both depend in part on the thyroid.

Biological time-keeping

A properly-working thyroid is of crucial importance during the developmental stages. It is the thyroid that 'tells' each part at the appropriate time when and how to grow, in accordance with the genetic blueprint provided by the parents. The unborn baby's thyroid goes into hormone production from about the third month of gestation, but the baby still requires a supply from his or her mother.

Birth is a dramatic event from any viewpoint, including that of the thyroid. As soon as the umbilical cord is cut, the baby's thyroid springs into action, flooding the bloodstream with its hormone. This very high level reaches a peak about the second day, and continues for six to eight weeks. Growth and development run at the maximum. It is because of the high metabolic rate induced by the thyroid, and the presence of brown fat, that tiny babies survive when adults perish. Babies buried under rubble in the 1985 Mexican earthquake lived without warmth or nourishment days after rescuers were abandoning hope of finding anyone alive.

Premature babies, however, do not have this remarkable thyroid reaction to coming into the cold world. They must have care in an incubator until their thyroid is sufficiently mature.

Throughout childhood the thyroid is concerned with growth and development, particularly of the bones and teeth and of the brain and nervous system. The timing of the first and second sets of teeth and how tall a child grows are of interest, but not of such vital importance as mental and emotional development. For children this includes behaviour, potty training and how they get on at school, in every way. An underactive thyroid is far more damaging than the overactive type, and today all babies in the West have their thyroid function checked at birth.

Problems arising later are less serious, and once recognized can be treated effectively.

At puberty, the thyroid is again actively involved in the changes from child to man or woman If a human adolescent is short of thyroid, he or she will look like a ten-year-old at seventeen – short and childlike, with undeveloped sexual organs. The secondary characteristics will be delayed too – breast development and periods for a girl, voice-breaking and the need to shave for a boy.

Women and the thyroid

The creation of the next generation depends on healthy thyroid glands in today's adults, especially the females. If the thyroid is either overactive or underactive, fertility plummets in either sex. In general, however, thyroid problems affect women much more often than men. A woman's metabolism is more complex and delicate than a man's. Oestrogen, the female sex hormone, makes women more responsive to the effects of thyroid hormone than men. Men's sex hormones – the androgens – have the opposite effect.

The ever-running female cycle of preparation in case of conception, then the period; the miracle of pregnancy and later of making milk, and the dramatic sign-off at the menopause are essential female concerns. Every one of them requires the correct thyroid input.

A woman's emotional system is also more susceptible to upset than a man's. Even minor thyroid disorders can bring on depression or an anxiety state in a woman, while men are affected only by serious thyroid dysfunction. There are two periods when a woman is particularly vulnerable, especially to emotional upset: after having a baby and at the change. At each of these times there is a sharp fall-off in the production of the female sex hormone, because of reduced need. At the same time there is a small reduction in the need for thyroid hormone. If the thyroid switches down too far temporarily, a new mother may be depressed, and low in energy. Similarly with a menopausal woman. If the thyroid keeps going normally, however, without much dip in output of hormone, the mother will be less likely to have a postnatal depression, and the fifty-year-old less likely to have the discomforts of hot flushes, low mood and weight gain. (Probably more women blame their thyroid for middle-aged spread, however, than are truly justified.)

Other stress

The thyroid interacts with the two stress hormones: cortisol, the body's own steroid, and adrenalin, the emergency hormone. Thyroid activity goes down when cortisol is called into play, but enhances the action of adrenalin. Thyroid hormone is also increased in response to the stress of taking an exam, or during a surgical operation: the metabolism of most tissues is increased, except in the brain.

What are the thyroid hormones?

The thyroid hormones are unique in containing iodine as a key ingredient: the gland takes what it needs from the circulating blood and within minutes converts it into a form in which it can be stored for use as and when needed.

A normal diet contains more than enough iodine to supply the thyroid. All it needs is about 1 milligram (1 mg) a week – a quantity too small to see. Iodine is present in various foods, tap water and milk. In some inland and mountainous areas there is a shortage of iodine in the soil, which can cause problems if the inhabitants produce all their own food locally. This doesn't apply in Western countries, since our food comes from many sources. Iodized salt is no longer considered necessary anywhere in the United Kingdom, though it is still available in the United States.

Too much iodine is as bad as too little. As with some vitamins, an excess is toxic, and particularly upsets the thyroid. It is unwise to take any extra unless your doctor specifically advises it.

Tweedledum and Tweedledee

The two major thyroid hormones are referred to as T_4 (thyroxine) and T_3 (triiodothyronine). Each chemical unit, or molecule, of T_4 contains four atoms, of iodine; each molecule of T_3 has only three. 90 cent of the thyroid output is T_4, 10 per cent is T_3. They both have the same stimulating effect, but T_3 is four times as powerful as T_4 and works eight times as fast.

The neat arrangement is that T_4 can turn into T_3 at the drop of a hat, by shedding one of its iodine atoms. This happens on site – that is, in the part, say your leg muscles, where an immediate boost to the metabolism is required. On the other hand there may be a call to reduce the metabolic rate – because of low fuel reserves due to slimming, or an illness that requires minimal use of the body's resources. In this situation there is an efficient shut-down of the slow T_4 and fast T_3 stimulating effects, by the conversion of T_4 into so-called reverse-T_3, which does not stimulate the metabolism.

Back-up arrangements

The thyroid keeps a store of iodine, tied on to big protein molecules, and also up to three months' reserve of almost-ready-to-use T_4. This is the same idea as those ready-prepared meals on the supermarket shelves that just need heating up when you want them.

How does the thyroid know how much hormone to make?

Like all the other hormone producers – the ovaries, testes, adrenals, pancreas, placenta and embryo – the thyroid comes under direct orders from the great coordinator, the pituitary. The pituitary transmits its own instructions by special, individual hormones – in the case of the thyroid, thyroid-stimulating hormone, TSH.

The pituitary itself comes under the direction of the highest authority of all: the hypothalamus in conjunction with the limbic system which is wrapped around it and which affects both the emotions and the automatic control of body functions. The hypothalamus is a sliver of brain tissue in the safest possible place in the centre of your head. It is your personal GCHQ, a great communications centre continuously monitoring information from all parts of the body, for instance a fall in your blood-sugar level or an itch in your right big toe. It collects and analyses the incoming information and sets off various reactions. Its purpose is to keep everything running steadily, for instance your temperature, modifying it by sweating or shivering if necessary; your water balance, your sleep–waking cycle, your periods; your blood chemistry; your sexual activity, etc.

As well as the input of practical information, every nuance of feeling – pleasure, guilt, fear or contentment – every hope and desire, short- or long-term, and also your (free) will is conveyed to the hypothalamus. It collates all the information – practical, imaginative and feeling – and programmes the pituitary by a super-fast hotline. The pituitary, tucked under the brain, then instructs the body's numerous departments and coordinates them all, like the conductor of a magical orchestra. Modern microchip technology is as nothing compared with the marvellous subtlety of the hormonal apparatus we all have.

The odd hormone

It was not until the 1970s that another hormone, nothing like T_3 and T_4, was discovered in the thyroid. Its name is *calcitonin*, because it helps to control the amount of calcium you have in your blood and your bones. It is given as a medicine in the treatment of Paget's disease, a problem affecting some elderly people, in which certain bones start enlarging. A blood test for calcitonin has also proved to be useful in providing an early warning of one type of cancer.

2

Enlarged thyroid

Swelling of the neck from an oversize thyroid has been known since history was first recorded. It has had a variety of names, including struma, botium, galagande, gongrona, choiron and the one that has stuck: goitre. For centuries it was considered an enhancement of beauty, probably because it so often occurs in girls in their teens and twenties.

Cleopatra is depicted with a goitre in a relief at Dendera, in the Nile Valley, while Rubens's charming painting of his sister-in-law, Susanna Fourment (*Le Chapeau de Paille* in the National Gallery, London), shows a pretty, sprightly young woman with a big hat and a noticeably large thyroid.

Like everything to do with the thyroid, goitre affects more women than men, but not exclusively. Around 1550 Michelangelo's surgeon pointed out for the first time that females in general have larger thyroid glands than men. Michelangelo himself was one of those men who develop a big thyroid. He drew a sketch of himself with the typical bulge at the front of his neck, in the margin of a sonnet he wrote for a friend, and annotated it 'I've grown a goitre by dwelling in this den . . .'. The 'den' was the Sistine Chapel, which was taking him a long time to paint.

There are in fact seven principal *types of thyroid enlargement*, which we will look at in turn:

1. normal, physiological;
2. simple;
3. multinodular;
4. nodular;
5. endemic – from iodine-deficiency and other chemical effects;
6. autoimmune – several types;
7. tumour – benign or cancerous.

Normal, physiological goitre

During adolescence
Throughout childhood there is no difference in appearance between boys' necks and girls'. That changes at puberty. When boys' voices are breaking and their larynx – Adam's apple – is

becoming more prominent, girls of the same age tend to a smoother, fuller look at the front of the neck, and it is quite common for there to be an actual bulge, or goitre. Most likely a friend or the doctor will be the first to notice it. Since there is neither discomfort nor tenderness and the youngster is perfectly fit, there is nothing to draw her attention to it.

The explanation lies in the teenage surge of the sex hormones into the circulation, particularly oestrogen in the case of a girl. The ovaries are coming on stream for the change-over to womanhood. Oestrogen has a stimulating effect on the thyroid. The thyroid responds by working harder to meet the increased need for hormones, and like a muscle after exercise, increases in size to an extent which may be noticeable. The gland does not produce more than is needed of its own hormones, so there are no general effects. None of this happens in boys growing up because male sex hormones – androgens – tend to have a damping-down effect on the thyroid (see Chapter 7).

Annabel was getting ready for her sixteenth-birthday party. As she clipped on the gold necklet she had been given the previous year, she was surprised to find it slightly tight. Looking at her neck in the mirror, she could see a distinct bulge which hadn't been there earlier. Then she remembered Aunty May, who had to have an operation for her thyroid. Annabel was scared and arranged to see her doctor. She was told not to worry, that in her case it was just a part of normal growing-up. She was to come back in six months for a check. Putting on the same necklet for her eighteenth-birthday celebration, Annabel found it was now comfortably loose again.

During pregnancy

Even more than during adolescence, in pregnancy there is an increased supply of oestrogen, and a need for greater thyroid activity to provide for the growing foetus. The gland often becomes measurably bigger. The Roman poet Catullus, in about 50 BC, described a state-of-the-art pregnancy test. A thread was tied round the woman's throat: if it became tight or broke, that was positive. The term 'honeymoon goitre' referred to the probability of pregnancy in the days before reliable contraception (see Chapter 5).

Other sources of extra oestrogen may mimic pregnancy and deceive the thyroid into doing extra work. They include the contraceptive pill and HRT (hormone replacement therapy). These may stimulate swelling of the thyroid. Cannabis acts similarly if used regularly.

Physiological enlargement of the thyroid does not usually persist after the rhythm of the periods is well established in an adolescent or, after pregnancy, when the new baby is six to eight weeks old. Sometimes, however, instead of reverting to its previous, undetectable, state, the thyroid remains big and may gradually get bigger. This is one type of simple goitre.

Simple goitre

This means enlargement of a healthy thyroid gland with neither over- nor under-production of thyroid hormones. The commonest form, worldwide, is the endemic type (see page 19). Omitting the endemic type, however, it has been estimated that around 5 per cent of people in the USA develop a simple goitre at some time in their lives. This may simply be a continuation of the physiological swelling of puberty or pregnancy, but it can also crop up out of the blue, affecting some men as well as women. The gland commonly enlarges to two or three times its normal size – which is still not very noticeable – though it may become huge.

The enlarged thyroid is smooth, symmetrical and soft to the touch. The likeliest age for it to appear is between fifteen and twenty-five, and there is a good chance of its returning to its earlier size over two or three years. It is unlikely to cause any problems, except possibly a slight feeling of tightness on swallowing at times.

What to do

The first step is to have a discussion with your doctor, so that he or she is aware of the situation. Unless he or she finds something else when examining you, treatment is unnecessary from the point of view of your health. If the bulge is annoying you by its presence, the doctor may think it worthwhile to give you a small daily dose of thyroxine (thyroid hormone) to encourage the gland to shrink down. This seems to help in some cases, but not all.

In the uncommon event that the goitre becomes unsightly or uncomfortable from its size, you may decide to have a tidying-up operation. This is more often required by older people with the multinodular type of goitre: below.

Multinodular goitre

This form may develop over ten or twenty years from a simple, smooth swelling that did not go away, but it can crop up out of nowhere and, unlike the simple type, it stays. The peak age range for it to appear is thirty-five to fifty-five. A mild degree of this condition is extremely common, probably affecting 60 per cent of middle-aged women, many of them unaware of it. Instead of being smooth like a cushion, the gland develops an irregular, lumpy consistency. This may be noticeable to the feel, and there is more or less enlargement.

The thyroid is still producing the appropriate quota of hormones, so there are no general symptoms. From around age sixty onwards there is a slightly greater likelihood of it causing local pressure problems. If there is pressure on the windpipe –tracheal compression – it can make breathing noisy at times, while slight pressure on the gullet can make it uncomfortable to swallow a hard chunk of meat, for instance.

Nodular goitre

This is the term used when there is only one noticeable lump or nodule in or on the thyroid, which is working normally. Usually there are other nodular parts which don't show.

Substernal goitre

Particularly where there is a single, sizeable thyroid nodule, this may grow downwards as you get older, say through the sixties. It may extend behind the sternum, or breastbone. This may not matter at all, or there may be a squash of tissues hemmed in by the bone. In that case there may be really troublesome difficulties in breathing and swallowing, often with wheezing and a hoarse voice, quite different from what it used to be like. The thyroid itself may continue to function normally.

What to do about multinodular and nodular thyroid

Tests While your doctor may be content to do nothing if you have a simple goitre and no problems, he is likely to want to run a few tests if you have developed the multinodular type, which usually persists. He will be even more interested in checks if there is a lot of thyroid trouble of any sort in the family. Blood tests will establish whether your thyroid is making the right amount of hormone, whether it is working under difficulties, and whether there are any antithyroid antibodies circulating (see autoimmune problems, page 23). Blood tests (see page 118) will also pick up other chemicals or organisms which might interfere with the harmonious working of the gland.

17

X-rays and scans In the case of pressure symptoms, X-rays are vital – plain, CT scan or barium swallow. For the last, a film is taken while you are swallowing a drink that shows up on an X-ray. This indicates any area of pressure on the gullet. The general size and outline of the thyroid shows in an ordinary X-ray, and ultrasound (see page 123) also gives a picture. If a substernal goitre is suspected, a CT scan, which produces pictures as though you were sliced across horizontally, reveals the exact situation at every level.

To check whether the nodules in a nodular thyroid are producing hormones normally, there is a special type of X-ray called a scintigram (see page 122). This is not usually necessary, but if there is just one lump it is especially important to make sure what it is. It may be a harmless cyst, an area of overactive thyroid tissue (a 'hot spot'), an adenoma, which is an unimportant irregularity, or – least likely – a cancer.

FNA – fine-needle aspiration (see page 123) – is a quick, painless way of taking a sample of the lump, called a biopsy, and finding out with a microscope its exact composition.

Treatment

If the tests show that your thyroid is working normally and its size is no bother to you, no action is needed at present, but you should have an annual check. If there were antithyroid antibodies in your blood, it is particularly sensible to have this follow-up. Your hormone production could fall off gradually without your being aware of it, even if it is satisfactory now.

Of course, if you are found to have too much or too little thyroid hormone your doctor will ask you a lot more questions and perhaps arrange further tests. Then you will start on definite treatment.

This is likely to be medication of whichever kind is appropriate (see Chapters 3 and 4). If, however, your thyroid is too bulky to be elegant and comfortable, if it is causing pressure problems in your breathing or swallowing tubes, or if it has sneaked behind your breastbone, an operation is the quickest, safest and most effective treatment. There is no medicine that will make an enlarged thyroid shrink when it has become nodular. On the other hand you will probably need to take thyroxine (synthetic thyroid hormone) indefinitely after the operation. This will not only prevent your running short of the hormone now you have lost part of the production line, it will also tend to discourage any propensity in the remaining part to overgrow again.

Where there is a single nodule of any kind – whether a harmless cyst, an overactive hot spot, a tumour or a substernal goitre – surgery is the best treatment.

Philip was thirty-eight. He managed the supermarket efficiently and was generally fit. He had sailed through a recent insurance medical. It was his wife who pushed him to see the doctor. We all choke at mealtimes occasionally, when something 'goes down the wrong way', but Phil did it often, especially when they were out. He had spells of coughing from time to time and insisted on three pillows.

The doctor could find nothing wrong physically, and thyroid tests were all normal, so he arranged a chest X-ray. This showed a fleshy lump behind the breastbone. A CT scan located it better, and a scintigram showed that it was active thyroid tissue – a substernal goitre.

The unwanted part of the thyroid was removed surgically, and the symptoms with it. The scar at the base of Philip's neck hardly showed, but had he been a woman he might have covered the thin line with a necklet.

Endemic or iodine-deficiency goitre

Everything we have discussed so far has been concerned with a healthy thyroid growing oversize without any apparent outside cause and continuing to function normally. There are various other conditions in which the thyroid swells up in response to something harmful to it. In iodine-deficiency goitre there is a clear cause from the environment.

Endemic goitre – so called because it is regularly found in certain regions – is still prevalent in many parts of Asia, Africa and South America, especially in such mountainous districts as the Himalayas and the Andes. It affects more than 300 million people in Asia alone. There are also a few isolated pockets in Europe, in the Alps, where there used to be goitre epidemics, but these are no longer a problem in the industrial countries apart from in exceptional circumstances.

All the places where iodine-deficiency goitres are found are distant from the sea, the basic source of iodine in the world. Iodine gets into the soil and the water supplies from the wind and the rain off the sea, and thence into the plants. From there it also gets into the milk and meat that people eat. As well as areas far away from sea breezes, some valleys which have been cleared of their topsoil in the long past by glaciers have been left bereft of iodine, even near the coast. South Wales is one such area. (The ancients thought the

19

reason some people developed goitres in the valleys was because the air was 'too concentrated' there.)

With our sophisticated transport and distribution systems in the industrialized countries, we get our food from all over the world: bananas from Belize, coffee from Colombia, oranges from Israel . . . and fish from the sea, too – another fine source of iodine. In the remote areas of the Third World only local produce is available, and its iodine content is dependent on the mineral content of the soil there.

If a Westerner takes a short trip to Tibet or a safari across Africa, he or she may be deprived of iodine because of the environment. This will not matter – remember the three months' reserve supply stored by the thyroid (see page 12). On the other hand, if you are planning to stay for months or years in a far-away mountainous district, it would be wise to check if goitre is prevalent there. Discuss with an expert the advisability of taking iodized table salt, for instance.

If you live in the West there is more danger of your taking too much iodine than too little. You cannot take too much from normal eating: the risk is in taking unprescribed iodine supplements, or becoming a kelp freak. Kelp is a seaweed which is very rich in iodine. It had a great vogue as a health food in Ancient China, medieval England and early-twentieth-century America, when goitre was rife in some states, such as Michigan. The thyroid responds to overdosing with iodine either by producing too much hormone or, paradoxically, by giving up. It enlarges either way.

The thyroid gland gets bigger when it has to work extra hard, as in pregnancy. Shortage of iodine – an essential constituent of the thyroid hormones – means that it has to manage under difficulties. In its efforts the gland swells up and may become enormous. Early pictures and descriptions of goitre are likely to be those of people living in iodine-deficient areas. The Chinese in 1600 BC and the Vedic Indians 1,200 years later, found a cure: powered burnt seaweed or sponge in wine. Later they found powdered mollusc shells equally efficacious. No one knew about iodine until centuries later.

Europe was slow to catch on, compared with Asia, although Hippocrates – 400 BC – noticed the association between goitre and mountains. He put it down to drinking melted snow. The Romans also blamed 'the noxious qualities of the water' in the Alps. Marco Polo, in his travelogue of 1299, described 'tumours of the throat, occasioned by the quality of the water'. No cure was mentioned.

In England, Shakespeare had Gonzalo in *The Tempest* speak of 'mountaineers . . . whose throats had hanging at them wallets of flesh'. In the eighteenth century most of the countries of Europe included particular 'goitre areas': the Tyrol, the West Pyrenees, the Bavarian Alps and, in England, Derbyshire. A 'Derbyshire neck' was a matter of pride – like a Yorkshire accent.

It was not until 1811 that Bernard Courtois discovered what he called 'Substance X', violet-coloured crystals. This was iodine. Over the next fifty years, despite disastrous mistakes in how to use it, iodine came to be the cure or preventive measure for endemic goitre. The Swiss were the first to have the idea of putting iodine in the salt people used; by 1917 they had eliminated the illness from their country. The Americans cottoned on soon after, but it was not until 1960 that the British caught up. Now, however, because of the variety of foods available to everybody, iodization is no longer necessary in this country.

Although lack of iodine in the soil is the main cause of endemic goitre, it is not the only one. The next great discovery about goitre can apply to any of us today. In 1928 Dr Alan Chesney at John Hopkins Medical School realized that something in cabbage was causing his rabbits to develop swellings in their necks. Now we know that the brassica group of vegetables – cabbage, kohlrabi, sprouts, cauliflower (but not broccoli) – contain goitrogens (see page 109). These are chemicals that prevent the thyroid from making its hormones in spite of plenty of iodine and produce an effect similar to that of iodine shortage.

In the case of brassica the goitrogens are cyanide derivatives called thiocyanates. They also come through in milk from cows who have been fed on kale and raw turnips which people do not eat directly. Children in Tasmania started developing goitres through drinking milk from kale-fed cows. This was most noticeable in the spring, when thiocyanate levels in the plants are at their highest. Other plants which have a similar effect include soya, oil-seed rape and peanuts (see page 109).

Among adults, only cranks are likely to consume enough brassica vegetables to develop goitres, but there are some commonly used medicines (see page 109) which can also lead to this type of thyroid swelling. They include:

- lithium, used in psychiatric illness;
- phenylbutazone, for arthritis;
- PAS, for tuberculosis;
- tolbutamide, for diabetes;
- beta-blockers, for high blood pressure;

- resorcinol, a skin disinfectant;
- steroids.

Some iodine-containing medicines may, paradoxically, act in the same way:

- amiodarone, a heart medicine;
- potassium iodide, an ingredient in some cough medicines.

It would require regular use of any of these medicines to have an effect.

The goitrogens are more likely to tip the balance towards putting a strain on the thyroid if a person is already vulnerable. This may be because of autoimmune antibodies (see page 35), a diet low in iodine, or a family prone to thyroid problems.

The time-hallowed idea that bad water was a cause of goitre has some basis in fact. In some areas an excess of calcium in the water prevents the proper use of iodine by the thyroid. This is most likely in limestone districts. In Derbyshire, for instance, people who drew their water from two particular wells were found to develop goitres. Pollution with urochrome from urine or sewage can also poison the thyroid, and has been responsible for some goitres.

Features of the endemic type of goitre

People of any age can be affected, but women at least twice as often as men. The swelling usually begins uniformly but becomes multinodular and it tends to go on enlarging slowly. Sometimes, although the gland is working flat out under difficulties, it may not be able to make enough T_4 and T_3. In that case all the symptoms and signs of too little thyroid gradually develop. They often include general sluggishness, weight gain, swollen legs and thinning hair, but there are many exceptions – see Chapter 3. The changes creep up so imperceptibly that they may well not be recognized as abnormal but put down to increasing age.

An even more serious threat arises in pregnancy. While the thyroid may be able to produce all the hormones that the mother needs for herself, it is less likely, working under difficulties, to cope with supplying a fast-growing foetus. It was because of this that in the goitre areas so many cretins were born – the technical term for people deformed and mentally retarded as a result of thyroid deficiency from before birth. The children were stunted in every way and grew up into thyroid-deprived adults, so there was a population of many people with goitres, including some retarded, and children who never developed properly.

In 1848 in Chiselborough, a village in Somerset, all 540 inhabitants had goitres, many were dull and slow, and twenty-seven had major intellectual handicaps. A combination of goitre-producing factors in the environment was responsible. Luckily, no other place in England was so affected, and by 1871 the disorder had subsided in Chiselborough. Such a horror could not strike now. Due to efficient testing of adults who develop goitres and routine thyroid tests for pregnant women and newborn babies, these human disasters are a thing of the past in our culture. They will also be banished from the Third World with the spread of medical knowledge and techniques.

What to do

If you are on one of the medicines, long-term, that can upset your thyroid it is essential to have regular checks to make sure that your thyroid is producing adequate amounts of hormone and that it is not having a serious struggle to do so. The TSH test (see Chapter 10) provides this latter information. You don't want to wait until the symptoms of thyroid deficiency sneak up.

Treatment

If the tests are normal you will need no active treatment, but regular follow-up. If your hormone levels are satisfactory but your TSH level is raised, the doctor may put you on a small supplement of iodine and/or a small dose of thyroxine, to help the gland out.

You will need special monitoring if you become pregnant (see Chapter 5).

If you test low for the thyroid hormones, the shortfall must be corrected with thyroxine, even if you have none of the indications of underactive thyroid (see Chapter 3).

Autoimmune disorders

While the most prevalent thyroid problem, worldwide, is endemic iodine-deficiency goitre, the commonest thyroid disorders in the industrialized West are all due to autoimmune disease. In autoimmunity the body mistakenly reacts against its own tissues, making antibodies in the blood to fight what it sees as enemies that should not be there, like bacteria. In the case of the thyroid, one or more of several antibodies may be produced against the thyroid's proteins. It is often when the immunity system is under attack from a virus, or in some cases from a drug to which it is sensitive, that it overreacts and makes antibodies against friends as well as foes. The propensity to do this runs in families, in the genes. People who develop a thyroid disorder may have relatives with other autoimmune ill-nesses, for instance rheumatoid arthritis, diabetes or vitiligo (a patchy loss of pigment in the skin), or suffer from them themselves.

If you are one of those who are especially prone to develop autoimmune problems, these are increasingly likely to come on as you get older. Your immunity system gets less efficient: it has already had a lot to contend with, with childhood illnesses, jabs for holidays abroad, etc.

In the struggle to keep going in the face of interference by antibodies, the thyroid may react in several different ways, leading to important thyroid illnesses:

- Graves' disease – the dramatic, overactive type;
- Hashimoto's disease, chronic thyroiditis – very common, and leading to thyroid failure and hypothyroidism or underactive thyroid;
- underactive thyroid, with or without goitre;
- many cases of 'simple' goitre;
- de Quervain's thyroiditis.

Any of these is likely to be accompanied by a goitre. Apart from in some cases of simple, uncomplicated goitre and de Quervain's disease, while the gland may be enlarged, the main features of the illness will be due to under- or over-production of the thyroid hormones. These are dealt with in Chapters 3 and 4.

De Quervain's thyroiditis

This disorder was first described by Felix de Quervain in the 1920s, but only in 1993 was it recognized as an autoimmune illness. The autoimmune reaction seems to be set off by a virus – sometimes the mumps virus. Like mumps (though uninfectious), de Quervain's thyroiditis comes in mini-epidemics. Unlike the slow, painless onset of the other thyroid problems, this comes on very rapidly, with sudden, painful swelling of the gland.

The pain may feel as though it comes from the teeth, the jawbone or even the ear, but touching the hard, tender thyroid settles the question. It hurts to swallow, laugh or nod your head, and you have a headache, aching in the muscles and a raised temperature.

The illness goes through two very different stages, each lasting several months, after the general feeling of acute illness has died down. The first stage is overactivity of the thyroid, when it is reacting with irritation. You are nervous, restless, and have a racing pulse. The second stage is underactivity, when the gland is tired from its exertions. You slow down and feel weary, cold – and constipated.

Treatment

There is no specific medicine to deal with the cause, but plenty to make you more comfortable. Steroids, such as prednisolone, are likely to cut the whole illness short, but you may find mild painkillers, like aspirin or paracetamol, helpful for the initial neck pain. You may need beta-blockers to calm down your heart rate and your mind, and possibly a small dose of thyroxine in the final stages.

The good news is that nearly always everything goes back to normal in the end, although Hashimoto's underactive thyroid – another autoimmune problem – affects a few long-term.

It is very rare indeed for the bigger germs – the cocci and bacilli – to infect the thyroid. If this does happen you may develop a thyroid abscess, but antibiotics are effective.

Tumours of the thyroid

Adenoma of the thyroid – a noncancerous tumour or cyst, like the harmless, lumpy areas in the breast that cause so much needless worry – tends to crop up from around thirty-five onwards. It is no health risk, but it is usually more comfortable to have it removed and end any anxiety. It is far commoner than thyroid cancer.

No one welcomes cancer, but there are three plus points for the thyroid type. Firstly, it causes so little trouble that it is frequently discovered only after the person's death from something quite unrelated. Secondly, of those that are diagnosed in life, over 90 per cent are curable. Thirdly, there is an effective early-warning system from a blood test.

The tumour starts off as a lump in the thyroid. That is why any solitary nodule in the gland merits checking out thoroughly, however unlikely it is to be a cancer.

This is one thyroid disorder that doesn't run in families, and there is no extra risk if you have a goitre, or any other thyroid problem.

Treatment

The cancerous lump is removed surgically, with as much of the surrounding gland as the operator thinks necessary. For some people, radioiodine (iodine made radioactive), in the form of a drink or capsules, is given as an extra precaution after surgery. In all cases, replacement therapy with thyroxine tablets is needed indefinitely, to compensate for the loss of thyroid.

3

Underactive thyroid

The trouble with an underactive thyroid is that you may not know you have one. An underactive thyroid means that it isn't producing enough of its hormones, T_4 and T_3, for your mental and bodily needs. The scientific name for this is hypothyroidism. 'Hypo' is Greek for 'under'. (It is rather confusing since hyper means the opposite, so that hyperthyroidism means an overactive thyroid.) Another term still in use for underactivity is myxoedema. This was dreamed up by a Dr Ord in 1877, and it refers to the puffy swelling ('oedema') of the skin in this condition.

Underactive thyroid is common, and probably more so than is recorded. Take a trip on a bus or a train and you are bound to see at least one hypothyroid person. It is at least fifteen times as likely to be a woman as a man, and she will probably be between thirty and sixty years old. Like depression, which often goes with it, hypothyroidism usually creeps up so slowly that you think it's 'just you', or 'only to be expected at your age'.

Sir William Gull, Queen Victoria's doctor who first linked the thyroid with some curious changes affecting mainly those around the menopause, described one of his patients in 1873:

> Miss B., after the cessation of the catamenial period [i.e. after the menopause], became insensibly more and more languid, with general increase in bulk. The change went on from year to year, her face altering from oval to round, like the full moon at rising . . . the voice guttural . . . the hands peculiarly broad and thick.

Miss B. did not wake up one morning with a swollen face, as you do with mumps. The changes due to an underactive thyroid are so gradual that your family and even your doctor may not realize what is happening. Sometimes a doctor you have not seen before will spot the disorder:

> When Phyllis was visiting her mother, who was in hospital with diabetes, she had a chat with the houseman. To her surprise, he seemed more interested in her health than in her mother's. He had noticed that Phyllis was plump, a little short of breath, and had some of the external features of hypothyroidism.

For most of us, neither the Queen's doctor, as in the case of Miss

B., nor a bright young ward doctor may cast a clinical eye over us. It is up to us to report to our doctors any changes, including the vague, general ones. Nowadays, unlike in 1873, it is extremely worthwhile to recognize thyroid deficiency as soon as possible, because there is a certain cure.

If, for instance your skin seems to be getting slightly thicker and yellowish, you've put on a few pounds without eating any more, and everything feels an effort, don't just assume it's your fault. One reason for the insidious way in which thyroid-deficiency problems come on is that the gland struggles to keep going in the face of difficulties, often getting bigger with the effort. Another reason is our big reserve store of both iodine and partly manufactured hormones.

What to look out for

Another factor that allows so many people to slip into hypothyroidism unawares is the extraordinary variety of symptoms it can produce, apparently with no rhyme or reason. You can't tell which is likely to affect you, nor in what order. They include three groups, those affecting:

- appearance,
- physical health,
- mental and emotional state.

Appearance

Any of the following features, in an early stage, may alert you to the possibility of an underactive thyroid. Comparison with a snapshot taken a few years ago can make any changes more obvious.

Face Full and puffy. The skin looks thick – almost padded – notably the eyelids, and especially the lower ones.

Complexion Pale and porcelain-like from anaemia, but with a pink flush over the cheekbones, or of a lemony tint. This is from a build-up of carotene in the body, because it cannot be converted to vitamin A without adequate thyroid hormone.

Lips Swollen and pouting, of a purplish hue. The colour is due to poor, slow circulation. The tongue is enlarged, and may be more visible than usual.

Eyebrows The outer third on each side lose their hairs.

Expression Sad, lack-lustre.

Head and body hair Becoming scanty and paler. There is no sheen on the head hair, so it looks as though it is dulled by too much hairspray. The hair will not hold a perm.

Skin Thick, dry and slightly peeling; cool to the touch. There may be a 'granny's tartan' rash over the body, like a reddish network.

Vitiligo A patchy loss of pigment in the skin, affecting any area, and slowly spreading over more of the body and face. It is made worse by the sun. Although it looks odd, the skin is perfectly healthy. This is an autoimmune condition.

Nails They are very slow-growing and develop ridges.

Xanthelasma This is the name for little yellow lumps round the eyes. They are made of cholesterol, and indicate a high level in the blood. They can be a useful hint to have a thyroid check, and in any case they are a warning to take steps to reduce the fat in your bloodstream.

Hands, feet and ankles They are enlarged, so your rings and your shoes are too tight.

Clothes These are as characteristic as any other outward feature of an underactive thyroid. You will be wearing thicker, heavier, woollier garments, and more of them than previously.

Physical health

Heartbeat The usual effect of hypothyroidism is a slowing of the heart rate, but the heart rhythm may also be put out, particularly in those over fifty. The rate may be as low as fifty beats a minute compared with the usual of seventy to eighty. A slow heart rate means sluggish circulation, in turn leading to cold skin, blue lips, ankle swelling, impotence and a risk of congestive heart problems. An uncorrected high level of cholesterol can result in furred arteries and the possibility of heart attack. Palpitations may occur.

Blood pressure This may be low because of the slow heart rate, or raised because of furring of the arteries with excess cholesterol.

Chest pain In people with Hashimoto's type of hypothyroidism (page 35), pain in the front of the chest is common. Angina, on the other hand, is uncommon when there is a low level of thyroid hormones, but if treatment is started too abruptly the typical chest pains of angina are likely to arise. Anginal pain feels tight and constricting across the chest when you are walking uphill, but stops when you do. This effect during thyroxine treatment is temporary, but requires a slow-down in building up to the correct dosage.

Shortness of breath This is common, and has several contributing causes, including increased weight, anaemia, slow heart and collection of fluid in the chest – similar to getting swollen ankles.

Weight The most typical change is a slow increase of, say, 10 lb over a year, despite a fall-off, if anything, in appetite. This is due to the slow rate of metabolism.

In 1947 Dr Adolf Magnus-Levy was studying obesity. He gave a fat nurse extra thyroxine, and found that she was using up 30 per cent more oxygen than before. He realized that this meant that she was burning up her food faster, and from this he developed the concept of basic metabolic rate (BMR – see Chapter 1), with the thyroid hormones setting the pace. The nurse had been hypothyroid, and she lost her excess weight gradually when her hormone levels were restored to normal.

Not all those who are short of thyroid hormones put on weight – some may actually get thinner, because their metabolism is inefficient in its slowness. This can apply at any age but is most usual in the over-thirty-fives.

Another anomaly that can spoil your figure is bloating – a build-up of wind during the day, making your tummy bulge. It isn't fat, and may be helped by a change of diet as well as by thyroid treatment.

Tinnitus This is an irritating ringing or whistling noise, usually in one ear only. It bothers two-thirds of those with an underactive thyroid. Unlike tinnitus resulting from other causes – wear-and-tear and damage – this type may improve with treatment.

Deafness This affects about one-third of those with an underactive thyroid; you find that you miss hearing the telephone sometimes. It is due to a direct effect on the hearing nerves (from a shortage of T_4 in the nerves), is seldom severe, and gets better with thyroid treatment.

Voice change This is due to swelling of the vocal cords and of the tongue, and it is most noticeable on the telephone. The doctor and philosopher Robert Asher described the effect as 'like a bad gramophone record of a drowsy, slightly intoxicated person with a bad cold and a plum in the mouth'. It doesn't often reach anything like that. You might at first find it rather sexy – your voice is a little deeper and huskier than usual.

Intolerance to cold Your internal heating is turned right down, so you feel unpleasantly chilly when everyone else complains of the heat. Your hands and feet are cold, and you are subject to chilblains or Raynaud's disorder. In the latter, your hands go mottled red and dead white at the slightest coolness, and are painful, blue and swollen when you warm them. You are at more risk than other people of developing hypothermia. Although thyroid treatment will put matters right, it takes several months to do so. During that time keep your home at 21°C.

Sleep You miss out on 'Stage-4' sleep – the deepest and most restful type. Loss of this leaves you tired all day, and sleepy.

Snoring Your partner will be more aware of this propensity than you, but you may also have 'sleep apnoea'. In this, your breathing slows down in your sleep, and then speeds up again with a jerk which may wake you up several times a night. You are unrefreshed and headachy in the morning.

Muscles In general they very gradually become weaker and stiffer, and they may ache. All of them may be affected, but especially your shoulders and thighs. It is difficult to keep up on a walk.

Cramp in the calves This may catch you when you are walking uphill, because of your poor circulation. Muscle cramps coming on even when you are resting happen only if your thyroid has been knocked out suddenly – for instance by an operation or by radioidine given without sufficient preparation, for overactive thyroid.

Joints Like your muscles, these too may be stiff and painful. They may be swollen by fluid in them. Those most likely to be affected are your knees, fingers, wrists and neck – or any one of them. Unlike with other forms of arthritis, the discomfort is not usually any worse in the mornings when you first get up. Thyroid treatment is effective, but it may be a year or more before full recovery.

Pins and needles There are two ways in which lack of thyroid hormone can cause this odd, unpleasant sensation in your fingers. The most likely is a direct effect on the nerves to your hand, but in about 7 in 100 it is a symptom of the 'carpal tunnel syndrome'. The carpal tunnels are the sheaths which cover the tendons in your wrists, and they may become swollen, like many other parts, in hypothyroidism. This makes it painful and stiff to move your fingers, as well as causing pins and needles.

Dizziness and poor balance These are also due to thyroid lack impairing the nerves. The unsteadiness can make you nervous about going out, but if it is a thyroid problem there is an answer.

Tremor Especially when you go to pick up a cup of tea. Like pins and needles, this may be because of shortage of T_4 to the nerves of your hands.

Faints Because of a slow circulation, leading to low blood pressure, these become more likely.

Periods They often become very heavy, and more frequent as well, but in a minority they stop altogether. There is also a general tendency to bleed for longer than usual if you cut yourself.

Infertility This is a common effect in either sex (see Chapter 5).

Anaemia You may develop either the ordinary iron-deficiency type, which is made worse by heavy periods, or pernicious anaemia. This is an autoimmune disorder like the Hashimoto type of underactive thyroid (see page 35), and you may develop the anaemia first.

Constipation This is particularly likely to be a nuisance to the older person. The cause is in the nerves controlling the bowels.

Don't think that you will suffer many or all of these physical symptoms, but if one or two of them crop up without an obvious reason, tell your doctor. Lack of thyroid hormones may not be to blame, but it is worth checking out since there is such an easy cure if it is.

With Marion it was the cholesterol that put her doctor on the track. The firm she worked for – an American company – was concerned to keep its executives on the top line, healthwise.

When everyone had to have a cholesterol check Marion's was found to be right in the risk range. At thirty-five and quite slim, this came as a shock. But there were other things. She had been feeling tired for some time and had wondered if it could be ME, or perhaps it was because her periods had been so heavy lately. Another problem was her stiff, aching neck and fingers, which she put down to keyboard work.

The thyroid tests showed that Marion was short of T_4, and examination told the doctor that the gland was slightly enlarged. Treatment restored her to the happy, lively, efficient young woman that she was naturally, with no aches or pains.

Mental and emotional state

In a way you are lucky if an underactive thyroid brings on physical disorders: it is much easier to mention these to your doctor than vague, intangible, psychological changes. For instance, how do you explain the paradox that, although you long to be warmer, you actually feel generally worse on a lovely hot holiday in the sun? This is because the heat switches down your already substandard thyroid production.

Changes in your outlook, feelings and efficiency that could indicate thyroid deficiency include the following:

- Sluggishness and apathy. You can't seem to care, even about people, and nothing catches your interest.
- Your senses of smell, taste and hearing are blunted, so that such pleasures as eating or listening to music are dulled too.
- A constant feeling of fatigue, although you are doing less than usual.
- Drowsiness all day and evening. You never see the end of a television programme because you drop off.
- Libido – your sexual feeling – is non-existent, however attractive your companion.
- Efficiency is well down.
- Your memory is unreliable, especially for recent events.
- Your concentration is poor – you can't cope with anything heavier than a magazine or newspaper article.
- Decisions are put off. Your mind goes round and round wearily getting nowhere.
- Day-to-day tasks seem outsize.
- Nothing feels right about yourself or anything else. This is the worst aspect, and you can't shake it off. The two main strands are depression and anxiety. Two-thirds of people with thyroid

deficiency suffer from depression, one-third with anxiety, often overlapping.

Depression includes pervading unhappiness, loss of hope, and the feeling that you are no good. You try to avoid other people, and wish you could go to sleep until the nightmare is over. Nothing is enjoyable. Appetite, energy and sleep are all reduced.

Anxiety results in your feeling agitated, sure something will go wrong and worried about things you would have taken in your stride before. You can't relax, but you can't get anything done.

Eddie was forty-three and his wife was fed up. They had been married fifteen years. They had no children, but, as Susan said bitterly, that wasn't surprising since they hardly ever had sex these days. Eddie was a big chap, with a fat face – not that he ate a lot – and he was bone-lazy. The slightest effort and he'd moan about being tired, in that irritating sloppy way of speaking that he'd developed.

Eddie worked for the electricity company, reading meters. It was when he kept making silly mistakes with the numbers, and missing some addresses altogether, that Susan got him to see the doctor. Perhaps he was run-down. The doctor saw at a glance the pale, puffy face and thick lips, the dry, cold skin, peeling slightly. His pulse was slow and his blood pressure low; otherwise there was nothing out of the way – not even a noticeable thyroid. Thyroid tests, however, showed that Eddie was well into the hypothyroid range. This was something that could easily be put right, although it took several months for the tablets to have their full effect.

If Eddie had been a housewife, the chances are that no one would have done anything.

Serious psychiatric disorder – psychosis

This is rare and arises only when someone has been short of thyroid hormone for years. Ultimately, in this situation, the victim may lose contact with reality. She, or less often he, feels puzzled and afraid and thinks that other people are her enemies. Sometimes she believes she can hear them plotting, or sees people and scenes which come only from her own mind. Her family will find her irrational and odd in her behaviour, and will realize that she is ill in some way. Thyroid treatment is needed urgently.

Other psychiatric disorders can be involved in hypothyroidism. For example, there is an increased risk of Alzheimer's disease in people whose brains have been starved of T_4 long-term. Thyroid treatment, if indicated by tests, is both a preventive and in some people a helpful remedy. The improvement sometimes occurs even when there is no positive test or other sign of thyroid deficiency. Similarly, some depressives with no symptoms of hypothyroidism, who are not responding to antidepressants, recover if thyroid hormone is added.

Some children with faults in their chromosomal make-up and intellectually impaired – including those born with Down's, Klinefelter's or Turner's syndromes – are particularly susceptible to autoimmune lack of thyroid. They blossom with treatment.

Myxoedema coma

This dangerous condition is fortunately very rare, but it can be the first event to draw attention to the sufferer's thyroid illness. It is the end-result of untreated hypothyroidism that has built up over the years. Independent-minded, elderly women living alone who 'don't want to be a bother to anyone' are the most at risk.

A cold snap is often the final trigger. The victim is found ice-cold and barely rousable; her temperature may be as low as 25°C, compared with the normal 37°C. Understandably, the condition is often mistaken for hypothermia. Alternatively some other illness, such as bronchitis or a urinary infection, may have been the final straw by making extra demands for thyroid hormone. Tranquillizers can have the same effect. Treatment is needed urgently, and, unlike hypothermia, more than gentle rewarming is required. It must be in hospital, and include steroid injections.

What to do

If you have even a vague, slight reason for suspecting that you or a member of your family might have an underactive thyroid, consult your doctor about a thyroid check. A simple blood test is all that is required to start with. It is good news if the thyroid turns out to be underactive: it may be that an easy treatment with tablets will revolutionize your strength, mental efficiency, mood and energy. The first step is to find out what is causing the gland to underfunction, then to plan treatment accordingly. For example, if your thyroid is inhibited by some medication you are taking (see pages 109–11), it is sensible to review the dosage of this, rather than immediately taking extra T_4.

Causes of an underactive thyroid

Autoimmune disorder is by far the commonest reason for under-activity of the thyroid in the industrialized world. It is increasingly likely as you get older, especially if there is any rheumatoid arthritis, pernicious anaemia or diabetes in your family. The presence of antithyroid antibodies in a blood test is the give-away, even if there is no visible sign of enlarged thyroid. When hypo-thyroidism develops apparently out of the blue it is probably due to an autoimmune reaction, and similarly when it crops up in someone with a simple goitre (see chapter 2).

Hashimoto's disease

In 1912 the thirty-year-old Dr Hakaru Hashimoto studied four middle-aged Japanese ladies. Each had a firm swelling in the neck and symptoms of sluggishness, weight gain and dislike of the cold. Dr H. was so diffident about his paper that he sent it to be published in Germany rather than at home in Japan. It wasn't until 1956, however, that a group of Americans worked out the autoimmune nature of the problem. Hashimoto's was the first illness shown to be due to antibodies made by the immune system against its own body tissues.

Hashimoto's thyroiditis is a cause of goitre in children from the age of ten, but is much more frequent in adults. Women are affected twenty times as often as men. Usually the attack on the thyroid by the antithyroid antibodies has been going on for many years before it is recognized.

Diana's story is typical. She had 'always' had a slight fullness in the neck. Her mother had noticed it when Diana was about eighteen. It did not lessen over the next two or three years, like the ordinary physiological goitre of puberty, but increased a little. Her neck felt soft and normal, and she was perfectly well. When she was coming up to thirty the mild swelling shrank a little, but it felt rather tender and uncomfortable. For a few weeks Diana felt generally tense, but then this feeling and the discomfort subsided.

What was happening was that the thyroid was at last reacting to the attacks by the antibodies by becoming inflamed – thyroiditis. A brief period of overactivity made her tense and restless, but after that Diana's thyroid swelling, although quite small, was firm and rubbery to the touch. Scar tissue had formed in it. Years went by, busy with career, marriage, children, until in her fifties Diana developed various minor health problems. The snag was that she hadn't the energy to do something about them, while her family wrote her off as middle-aged.

Her 'rheumatism', shapeless figure, slight deafness and poor memory, plus an irritating habit of going to sleep over the TV and even at the theatre, didn't seem to add up to an illness. But her thyroid had finally been overwhelmed by the enemies from within and could no longer provide an adequate supply of hormones.

Her GP got on to the problem when Diana alarmed her family by having a couple of faints, and they called him in.

Diana could have had any of the varied symptoms of hypothyroidism. The trick is to be alert to the first hints, and report them to the doctor. This is particularly important if you are aware of having a goitre, but it may be small and insignificant. If it is large, a Hashimoto goitre often feels oddly heavy in the neck, unlike simple goitre.

While Hashimoto's is the most important cause of damage to the thyroid which prevents its working properly, there are others:

Iodine deficiency

This is seldom a problem in the West (see page 11).

Surgery

A thyroid operation for any reason may leave the gland depleted of active, hormone-producing tissue. A handful of surgeons in the 1880s noticed that, some time after being operated on for goitre or overactive thyroid, their patients developed what they called 'cachexia strumipriva'. This comprised the same collection of symptoms as myxoedema, and was a clue to the connection between the latter and the thyroid.

Nowadays surgeons try to leave enough thyroid for it to function, and also check their patients' blood for adequate amounts of thyroid hormones. About 20 per cent of patients need T_4 supplements after surgery.

Radioidine and other antithyroid drugs

While surgery is no longer the only treatment for an overactive thyroid, the medicines used instead may be even more destructive of thyroid tissue. Radioiodine is an excellent form of treatment (see pages 129-31), but its effects continue for years after it has dealt with the overactive disease. After one or two decades, between 65 and 70 per cent of those given radioiodine slip into thyroid deficiency and need supplemental T_4.

The other antithyroid drugs used to treat an overactive thyroid, such as carbimazole (Neo-Mercazole), methimazole (Favistan), or propylthiouracil (Propycil) have a similar effect, but quicker. This unwanted effect is usually reversible if and when the medication is no longer necessary, or fine tuning may be done by adding thyroxine as necessary.

Less common causes of an underactive thyroid include the following:

De Quervain's thyroiditis (see page 24) The aftermath of this more acute inflammation of the thyroid may be long-term damage to the active tissues. Complete recovery is the likelier outcome, but thyroxine treatment is needed until the gland can make enough hormone itself.

Excess of iodine This can arise from such medicines as amiodarone and potassium iodide (see page 111), cranky overuse of seaweed preparations (common in Japan – see page 108), or taking iodine supplements without the doctor's say-so. Too much iodine can stimulate the thyroid to make too much T_3 and T_4, or, conversely, can inhibit the manufacture altogether.

After giving birth Some mothers develop temporary thyroid failure, and require treatment while the phase lasts (see Chapter 5).

Lithium This substance is taken over an indefinite period as a preventive in some types of psychiatric illness. In some people it precipitates the autoimmune reaction Hashimoto's disease. Replacement thyroid hormone must be taken while a change is made to a different medication for the psychiatric condition. Over a third require this.

Other medicines which can impair thyroid function These include phenytoin, sulphonamide, tolbutamide, androgens, salicylates and steroids (see Chapter 10).

Diet This can be harmful in several ways (see Chapter 10):

- goitrogens in the food (see page 109) – vegetables of the brassica family, soya beans, almonds, sweet corn, and milk from animals fed on certain fodder – may inhibit thyroid functioning;
- an excess of fibre may cause the bowel to be emptied too soon for sufficient iodine to be absorbed;

● a strict salt-free diet may prevent the uptake of iodine.

Certain minerals in excess Cobalt, fluorine, calcium, bromine, nitrates – either from the water supply or from misuse of health foods, medicines or multivitamin/multimineral pills.

Starvation from any cause The most likely is the self-chosen type, anorexia nervosa (see Chapter 7).

Physical illnesses not related to the thyroid Any severe illness, and some that are not particularly severe, can cause an upset in thyroid production:

● liver disorders such as cirrhosis, physical damage and auto-immune liver disease;
● kidney disorders, such as nephrosis and chronic renal failure, which is accompanied by goitre in nearly half the sufferers. A kidney transplant causes the thyroid function to return to normal, but dialysis has no such effect;
● diabetes, but only if badly controlled with the occurrence of 'hypos';
● all cancers, but especially lung cancer;
● autoimmune diseases, especially pernicious anaemia, lupus, rheumatoid arthritis and Addison's disease (see pages 35 and 47).

There is a flash increase in thyroid production during a surgical operation, but in the convalescent period there is temporary hypothyroid stage. This also happens after a severe burn, but neither case needs treatment.

Drugs Those who use heroin or methadone illegally, and so without supervision, may inadvertently upset their thyroid.

Secondary hypothyroidism

All the problems mentioned so far have been due to the thyroid itself, and its reactions to various outside influences. In a few rare cases, however, thyroid-hormone deficiency can occur although the gland is in perfect working order and there is nothing in the outside environment upsetting it. Such cases are due to faults in the control centres in the pituitary gland and the hypothalamus (see page 12). These faults are of overriding importance in themselves, with thyroid problems secondary. A pituitary tumour, probably non-malignant, is the commonest of this rare group.

Treatment of an underactive thyroid

In essence, treatment of thyroid deficiency could not be more straightforward: simple replacement in tablet form of the missing hormone. This is all that is required in the vast majority of cases, but it is vital to eliminate or deal with any underlying cause also.

It was a marvellous breakthrough when Dr Murray, one of the first to believe that the thyroid affected every part of the body and brain, in 1891 cured his myxoedematous patient with injections of sheep thyroid. She lived a further twenty years, to the age of seventy-four, but it took the thyroid glands of 870 sheep to keep her in health. The next advance was finding that the extract was just as effective when taken by mouth. On Christmas Day 1914, another leap forward came when the chemist Edward Kendall discovered how to make pure thyroxine, such as we use today. Henceforward no sheep but a chemical process was all that was needed, and the product could be given in precise doses.

Although the thyroid produces two hormones – T_4 (thyroxine) and T_3 (triiodothyronine) – replacement is completely satisfactory with thyroxine alone, since the body converts T_4 to T_3 in the ordinary way, as and when needed. The usual dose of thyroxine ranges between 100 and 200 micrograms (mcg) daily, with proportionately more for children and less for the elderly. This is to do with growth and energy requirements.

Caution: it is important, if you are over forty-five or severely hypothyroid, to start treatment with a low dose, say 25 mcg daily or on alternate days. Your doctor will increase this in small steps over weeks and months. It is not worthwhile to test your thyroid status until two months after you have started the treatment. The final dose will depend on how you feel as well as on the test results.

Some people have harmless palpitations when they first take thyroxine. A small dose of a beta-blocker (see page 128) will tide them over the uncomfortable phase, which is temporary and not dangerous. Other people get aching in the muscles, which is similarly temporary, and of no serious significance. Indications that the dose is too high too soon are muscle cramps, angina, shortness of breath or ankle swelling. It is a matter of adjustment.

There is danger and no advantage in taking more T_4 than the tests and your doctor suggest. Rather like alcohol, the right amount is a good thing, but too much is bad.

Treatment must continue for life in most cases, being monitored from year to year by testing. A particular convenience is that there is no need to take thyroxine more than once a day, and it doesn't matter at what time.

The treatment of underactive thyroid is one of the most rewarding. Sir William Osler in 1896 was almost lyrical: 'that we can today restore children otherwise doomed to helpless idiocy and that we can restore to life the hopeless victims of myxoedema is a triumph of experimental medicine'. It is no longer experimental.

Metabolic insufficiency

There is a condition that causes a mix of vague symptoms which suggest thyroid deficiency despite a normal test result. It has been named 'metabolic insufficiency', and sometimes 'borderline hypo-thyroidism'. The signs are:

- lassitude and loss of interest in everything;
- everything is an effort – you are tired before you begin;
- mild anaemia – your doctor may just advise stepping up the iron-containing foods;
- constipation;
- feeling the cold;
- irregular periods;
- weight creeping up;
- hair thinning.

Treatment

Often you feel much better after starting on thyroxine, but the effect is only temporary unless you keep upping the dose. In the end even big doses don't work, and they throw a dangerous strain on the heart. This progression shows that, whatever else, the symptoms are not due to lack of thyroxine.

If missing a single dose of thyroxine makes the symptoms worse, and if there is a rapid improvement when you take the tablet, you are fooling yourself with faith. Thyroxine takes days to act – take it on Monday and it begins to have an effect on Friday. Conversely, missing a dose has no effect on the blood level of the hormone.

The symptoms you suffer are real enough, but thyroid tablets are not the answer. It's much more likely that some things in your lifestyle are undermining your health and happiness. You will need time and understanding to sort out what it is that is preventing your functioning at 100 per cent.

4

Overactive thyroid

'A lady, aged twenty, became affected by some symptoms which were supposed to be hysterical . . .' Dr Robert Graves was describing a patient in 1835. After about three months she developed a rapid heartbeat and a slight swelling of the front of her neck. These put him onto the idea that her problem wasn't 'all in the mind'.

It was similar for Katie. She was coming up to thirty and she and Harvey were planning to start a family. They'd had no luck so far, but they'd only been trying for a couple of months. Harvey put her snappishness down to frustration about that. Katie had always seemed easygoing, but now she blew up at the slightest thing, and she was so fidgety. Then she made a scene when her mother-in-law made a perfectly harmless remark. Harvey blamed Katie. She decided to ask the doctor for a tranquillizer.

He found she had a racing pulse and had lost about half a stone since Christmas, without trying. Katie was pleased about that, but went on to explain that she felt worn out for no special reason, and wasn't sleeping properly. Routine blood tests tracked down Katie's problems to an overactive thyroid. Unlike the situation for Dr Graves' patient, when the only treatment was blood-letting or purging, Katie's doctor was able to offer her a choice of genuine remedies.

The other names for overactive thyroid are 'hyperthyroidism', meaning excess of thyroid, and 'thyrotoxicosis', meaning poisoning by the thyroid.

An overactive thyroid usually reveals itself faster than the underactive type, but even so it is likely to be several months before the symptoms become so troublesome that you do something about them. As with most thyroid disorders, women are affected more often than men – eight times more often. There is no age limit in either sex, but if you have an overactive thyroid you are probably over twenty and under sixty. For the commonest kind of over-activity, you are especially vulnerable if there are any autoimmune diseases in your family (see page 47).

Just as in the case of an underactive gland, it is up to you to be the detective, and go for a check if you get a clue, however offbeat, that

41

your thyroid isn't working properly. The snag is that any system of your body, or your mind, may be the first to show signs of damage. It took the medical profession right into this century to work out the connections.

What to look out for

Mood   General nervousness, a mix of anxiety and irritability. You are liable to fly off the handle or dissolve into tears at the drop of a hat. It is like PMT all the time, only worse, even if you are past the change. You'll feel out-of-sorts but can't relax, and tired but can't sleep. You lie awake with thoughts rushing through your head and your heart thumping. What makes it worse is finding your bed unbearably hot. A few older people don't get the anxious mood: they react to the extra thyroid by an absence of any feeling – complete apathy.

When it is your spirits and emotions that are most obviously out of order, you are at risk of being written off as neurotic. You are not. To quote an eminent Victorian, an overactive thyroid is 'a medical misadventure that might befall anyone'.

Tremor   This, too, may come over as neurotic, although it is a direct physical effect through the nerves. You may find your cup and saucer rattle embarrassingly, or your writing has become untidy-looking. Even worse is the internal tremor – your body feels trembly and uneasy inside.

Heart and breathing   Everyone with an overactive thyroid has some change in the action of the heart, and in the over-fifties this is usually the most important problem. At any age you are likely to have palpitations, an uncomfortable awareness of the thumping of your heart. Your pulse rate may be double the normal, at 150 beats a minute, and occasionally so strong that you can hear it.

The high speed and high pressure may not allow the blood to return to the heart efficiently between beats. This leads to swollen ankles and sometimes a collection of fluid in the chest (see Chapter 8). Since your heart is going at a rapid rate all the time, it cannot speed up when you make an effort, so you are liable to get short of breath. If you have asthma, that will get worse.

One of my colleagues at hospital who prided himself on his squash was mortified to find he was losing his edge – at twenty-nine. He became hopelessly out of breath even when he was playing the boss. It wasn't until he drove everyone to complain, by opening all the windows when it was arctic outside, that the penny dropped. He had an overactive thyroid.

Digestive system   You may notice early on, like Katie, that you have magically lost 7 to 10 lb, although you have been eating more than usual. You may also have a yen for those cold, sweet drinks which are so calorific. Some older people lose their appetite instead of feeling hungrier, and together with the weight loss this may make them worry unnecessarily lest they have some serious disease.

Your bowel movements will be more frequent than usual, and the motions may be pale from extra fat being rushed through before being digested. At the other end, your stomach may be irritable so that you easily vomit. This can become an urgent problem.

Skin   You are likely to perspire more, so that your skin is soft, warm and damp. The palms of your hands may look flushed, and little spidery veins may appear on your cheeks. The bonus is an ironing out of any wrinkles, but unfortunately this is not permanent. You may feel itchy all over, and hot, so that if you've booked a holiday in the sun you'll wish it had been Iceland.

In some people with the autoimmune type of overactive thyroid the skin changes colour. It may either go a shade darker all over, or, as in Hashimoto's disease, the curious patchy condition called vitiligo may develop – see page 28.

There are also two rare skin conditions which occur only in autoimmune thyroid disorder. You may get ugly patches of thick red skin over your shins and feet, or a podgy thickening of the skin of your fingers and feet, so that you can't get your rings on and off and your shoes are too tight.

If you notice that you bruise easily, this is likely to be due to the anaemia which occasionally develops: tell your doctor.

Hair and nails   Your hair may become extra fine and soft, with an increased tendency to go grey and an obstinate refusal to take a perm. It may also become thinner. In underactive thyroid the hair also becomes sparse, but it is coarse and brittle.

A curious sign of overactive thyroid is a partial loosening of the nails, so that the tips ride up slightly and can catch, for example in your tights when you are pulling them on.

Neck   Your thyroid gland may look and feel larger, to you or your doctor, but it may not be swollen at all if, for instance, the problem is too big a dose of thyroxine by mouth, for some other condition.

Muscles and joints When there is too much thyroid hormone circulating, it tends to speed up the normal breaking-down of the muscle fibres to a rate faster than they can be replaced. The muscles become weaker, and this is especially noticeable in the thighs and shoulders. Frozen shoulder, often on both sides, is common in hyperthyroidism. The painful stiffness is due to inflammation of the covering of the shoulder joint. Other joints are not affected, but sometimes there is a shoulder–hand syndrome: as well as the stiff shoulders, the hands may be swollen and painful.

It always seems surprising that antithyroid treatment should help this kind of problem, and that somewhat similar symptoms in people with an underactive thyroid should respond to extra thyroxine.

Sex You may find you've lost interest, but this isn't permanent. If you are a man you may not be able to perform, while for a woman it means scanty periods or perhaps none at all. You might wonder if you are pregnant, but you are not likely to conceive. If you do, there's an increased risk of miscarriage. For either sex, fertility is reduced.

Eyes Although they are by no means inevitable, eye symptoms are a particular characteristic of an overactive thyroid. Unusually, in thyroid matters, in this case men are more susceptible than women, as are smokers of either sex. Oddly enough, the eye problems can come on months before any others, or at the height of the illness, or after everything else has recovered. In most cases both eyes are affected, but the symptoms are mild. They amount to a gritty feeling, as though sand had blown into your eyes, and the eyes are uncomfortable in bright sunshine.

You may notice in a mirror, or a friend may point out, that your eyes look as though you are staring in amazement all the time. They seem bigger because the lids are drawn back and more of the white part of your eye shows.

In the autoimmune type of hyperthyroidism, Graves' disease (as occasionally in Hashimoto's disease – see Chapter 3), more serious eye changes may occur. Inflammation of the tissues behind the eyes pushes them forward. This is called 'exophthalmos', and another name for Graves' disease is 'exophthalmic goitre'. The swelling from the inflammation interferes with the drainage of tears: your eyes water, the upper lids become puffy, and bags form under the lower lids. You may find it difficult to look up, because of weakened eye muscles. This is tiring, and you may ache all round your eyes. At worst, without treatment there is a risk to your sight.

The eyes react badly to sudden changes, so treatment of the thyroid problem has to be started gently and carefully – see page 134.

What to do

The commonest symptoms of an overactive thyroid are a rapid heart, weight loss and a swelling in the front of the neck. There's no guarantee that you'll have any of these and, on the other hand, any one of the problems described in this chapter can be caused by some non-thyroid disorder, which may be important or trivial. What is certain is that an untreated overactive thyroid is dangerous. Before there was effective treatment, 25 per cent of sufferers died. If you suspect that your thyroid could be out of order, see your doctor for a check.

This consists of a physical examination and a blood test. The physical includes assessment of any thyroid enlargement, looking for skin or eye problems, and checking for tremor in your outstretched hands or your tongue. The doctor will count your pulse and listen to your heart. He or she may also listen over your thyroid for 'bruit' (see page 48) and try your reflexes, which are likely to be brisk and jumpy.

The essential adjunct to this examination is a blood test to measure your thyroid hormones. Other investigations are usually needed only in special circumstances. They include looking for antibodies, X-ray, scintigram, electrocardiogram, and measuring the protrusion of the eyes (see Chapter 11).

If the examination indicates that you are hyperthyroid, the next step is to decide why.

Causes of an overactive thyroid

An overactive thyroid may be due to faulty antibodies (i.e. an autoimmune disorder), as in:

- Graves' disease;
- toxic multinodular goitre (overactive lumpy thyroid);
- toxic nodule (one overactive lump);
- Hashitoxicosis (a stage in some cases of Hashimoto's disease);
- a stage in de Quervain's thyroiditis.

Other causes are:

- excess of iodine;
- excess of thyroid hormone by mouth;

45

- T_3 toxicosis, due to excess T_3 rather than T_4;
- disorder of the pituitary gland;
- cancer.

These different types of overactive thyroid require different management, and so do particular groups of people:

- babies (Chapter 6);
- children (Chapter 7);
- pregnant women and new mothers (Chapter 7);
- the over-fifties (Chapter 8).

Graves' disease

90 per cent of thyroid overactivity is due to rogue antibodies, and three-quarters of this autoimmune disorder is due to Graves' disease. This is named after Dr Robert Graves, a Dublin physician, with one of whose patients we opened this chapter. She was one of three women each with swelling in the neck and 'violent palpitations'. Graves wasn't the first to describe the condition – it has also been called Parry's, Flajani's and Basedow's disease, but their names never caught on.

Dr Caleb Parry gave a dramatic account of something that happened in 1786:

> Elizabeth S., aged 21, was thrown out of a wheelchair in coming fast down a hill . . . and was very much frightened though not much hurt. From this time she has been subject to palpitations of the heart and various nervous affections. About a fortnight after, she began to notice a swelling of the thyroid gland.

Apart from the swelling, which may not always be noticeable, today we would probably put Elizabeth's problems down to PTSD –post-traumatic stress disorder – the currently fashionable diagnosis. The idea that serious stress can stimulate thyroid overactivity was generally accepted until well after the Second World War. It seemed to be confirmed by a Danish experience. During the German occupation from 1942–44, the annual number of new cases in Denmark jumped by 300 per cent, to revert to the pre-war norm in 1945.

In 1956 Hashimoto's condition of underactive thyroid (see page 35) was recognized and proved to be caused by antibodies made in error by the immune system. Only a year later it was established that Graves' disease was produced in a similar way, but with different antibodies, including one known as TRAb. The long-accepted theory that an emotional shock or severe persistent stress had a direct effect on the thyroid was thrown out of the window as superstitious nonsense. Since then it has become clear that it is the immune system that is thrown out of gear by emotional upset, for instance bereavement.

Now it seems that stress is one of the triggers of the autoimmune process responsible for Graves' disease. You have to be a special sort of person to be susceptible. For example, you are likely to have a particular type of tissue, called HLA-DR3, as part of the biological make-up you inherited through your genes. That is why a propensity to Graves' disease and other autoimmune problems runs in families. The other autoimmune disorders which may be associated are:

- vitiligo – a patchy loss of skin pigment;
- pernicious anaemia – a weak state of the blood connected with lack of vitamin B12;
- rheumatoid arthritis – in the fingers and knees especially;
- diabetes – deficiency of insulin, controlling sugar in the blood;
- Addison's disease – a disorder of the adrenal gland, leading to general weakness;
- lupus – a skin and general disorder;
- polymyalgia rheumatica – many painful muscles;
- giant cell arteritis – a painful disorder which affects the temples;
- myasthenia gravis – a rare, severe muscle weakness;

and, unexpectedly,

- dyslexia – a reading or spelling difficulty, often involving transposing of letters.

If you or your family have any of these problems, you are more susceptible to Graves'. If any relative has the illness, that increases the risk – up to 50 per cent if it is your identical twin. If you are female, you run ten times the risk of a male. Graves' can crop up at any age from five upwards, but is especially likely at around forty – usually before forty in the UK, after forty in the USA. Hyperthyroidism may have different characteristics in the young, the elderly and after having a baby, but the commonest cause in all cases is Graves' disease.

There are no specific precautions you can take to avoid the illness, since you cannot change your sex or your genetic make-up, nor escape the unexpected disaster. You can look after your general health, however, and report any doubtful symptoms promptly (see Chapter 10).

Making sure it is Graves' disease

These are the special points your doctor will look for to distinguish Graves' disease from other forms of hyperthyroidism:

- The thyroid gland is always swollen, perhaps so slightly that you don't notice it yourself. It feels smooth and fleshy, and equal on both sides.
- Sometimes the gland is so active that it requires a greatly increased through-put of blood. If your doctor listens through a stethoscope, he or she will hear a soft 'shush-shush' sound. This is called 'thyroid bruit', and doesn't occur in any other condition.
- A racing heart, of which you are conscious, is always present.
- Nerviness and jangled emotions trouble 99 per cent of Graves' sufferers.
- Tremor is almost as common.
- Serious eye symptoms and patches of thickened red skin on shins and fingers crop up less often, but these symptoms only occur in Graves' disease.

Tests which confirm the diagnosis   Usually all that is needed is the standard 'thyroid screen' of blood tests, but additional antibody tests can be made, while a scintigram shows the gland is very active all over (see Chapter 11).

How to get well

If Graves' disease has been confirmed as the cause of your problems, this is the go-ahead to start treatment. In general, you need plenty of rest and nourishing food, and you and your doctor will decide between you which of the specific treatments will be best for you. This depends on your age, sex, size of goitre and personal circumstances. There are a number of choices. First there are two types of short-term treatment for swift relief of symptoms:

Beta-blockers These medicines, of which the best-known is propanolol, are often used for high blood pressure. They slow down the heart, relieving palpitations, make you perspire less, stop any tremor, and reduce your anxiety. You can take them two or three times a day or in a long-acting, once-a-day tablet.

Beta-blockers are a useful general-purpose starting treatment, since they act quickly and do not stay too long in the system when you want to stop them. The downside is that they have no curative effect – they merely suppress some of the symptoms – you must not take them if you have asthma, and when you stop them you must tail off gradually.

Iodine drops or tablets These switch off excess thyroid activity within a few days, but their effect wears off in about three weeks. They are used mainly in the run-up to a thyroid operation.

The longer-term curative treatments are as follows:

Antithyroid drugs These have a two-fold beneficial effect: they interfere with the overproduction of thyroid hormones and also suppress the underlying autoimmune process. The best known are carbimazole, methimazole and propylthiouracil (PTU), the first being favourite in the UK, the last in the USA. Whichever you are on, it takes two or three weeks to work, and while you are on it you need to have regular checks from your doctor. The dosage of the medicine varies with the severity of the illness and its progress. If the antithyroid drug is pushing you towards making too little T_4 and T_3, it is usually better to make up the deficit with thyroxine tablets rather than try to get the antithyroid dosage exactly right.

Most people have to stay on these tablets for eighteen months to two years, when there is a 40 per cent likelihood of a permanent cure, but your doctor may decide to try you without the medicine after any period over six months. Your thyroid may have settled back to normality, but if the symptoms creep back after a month or two it is no good going back on the medicine – you would be certain to relapse again.

Antithyroid tablets are the best treatment for children and adolescents, still developing, and they are often tried in young women up to the age of forty but they cannot be taken in the last month of pregnancy or during breast-feeding. Men in particular find the regular follow-up appointments irksome. For them and for those in whom antithyroids have not produced a cure, there are two major treatments available: radioiodine and surgery.

Radioiodine This is the treatment of choice for an overactive thyroid. Iodine that has been made radioactive is, naturally, taken up by the thyroid cells just like ordinary iodine, so its radioactive effect is concentrated in the gland. It was first used to cure Graves' disease in 1940 – a bonus from the research towards the atomic bomb. Radioiodine soon became the most popular treatment and has remained so. You take it by mouth, in capsules, usually on one occasion only. The thought of swallowing something radioactive sounds alarming, but over the last fifty years radioiodine has proved safe as well as effective. The only ill-effect is a slight soreness of the neck for the first few days.

The only precautions are for the sake of other people, and are temporary. The radioactivity that is not taken up by your thyroid will be eliminated in your water, mainly in the first two or three days, but until then you have to keep your distance from other people. That is, don't spend hours and hours very close to another adult, especially someone younger than forty – for instance in bed. For up to fourteen days (you will be told precisely how long), don't kiss anybody, and don't get any nearer than two yards from babies and children. Travelling by public transport is all right, but postpone any long journeys by car for a fortnight. After this period is over, you needn't worry about the radioactivity any more. The exception is pregnancy – best postponed for six months after taking the dose. Nor should you have this treatment during pregnancy (see Chapter 5).

The beneficial effects of radioiodine are permanent, but they don't come on full strength for about three months. A beta-blocker is a handy way of keeping you comfortable meanwhile. Over the ensuing ten to twenty years, there is a fair chance of your thyroid becoming underactive. This is easily put right with thyroxine tablets. You don't have to wait for any of the symptoms of thyroid-deficiency to develop: tests done at your annual follow-up will give your doctor advance information, and treatment can be started in good time.

Surgery An operation to remove part of your thyroid gland is the other choice for a permanent cure. It can be dangerous to do the operation on an overactive gland, however: it needs quietening down first. Beta-blockers only suppress the symptoms – a fast pulse for instance – but iodine and antithyroid medicines both act directly on the thyroid. For the best results, you take an antithyroid for a month and add iodine for the last ten days before the operation.

Most people opt for radioiodine nowadays, but surgery is the treatment of choice if you have an unsightly goitre or uncomfortable pressure symptoms, or if you are allergic to antithyroid drugs. You may also choose an operation if you think you might be pregnant, or want to be as soon as possible (see Chapter 5).

Men often go for surgery because of its speedy effectiveness, certainty and permanence, and they are less likely to worry about the scar than women. Usually the scar hardly shows, lying in a fold of the neck, and in men it is under the collar-and-tie area. The operation involves about a week in hospital.

Special areas of treatment

Eye problems The usual mild eye discomfort normally settles with soothing hypromellose drops and dark glasses – and of course no smoking, at least until the thyroid itself has recovered. Troublesome eye symptoms may improve if a beta-blocker is added to other treatment. While most eye problems improve in step with the thyroid itself, sometimes the timing seems unconnected. If you are unlucky enough to develop very protruding eyes, as well as experiencing discomfort you may see double. Steroid medicines are helpful, and if all fails cosmetic-type surgery can put matters right, or the more recently introduced radiation therapy.

Thickened patches of skin These may feel heavy, itchy and irritable, but the main problem is that they make your legs ugly and misshapen – or your hands. The most effective treatment is a steroid cream applied at night under something like clingfilm. You must be persistent and patient, maybe for over a year, to achieve a cure.

Toxic multinodular goitre

This autoimmune overactivity disorder is the second commonest, accounting for 14 per cent of hyperthyroidism. Like Graves' disease it affects many more women than men, but later – often at around age sixty.

Rita was typical. She'd had a mild fullness of the neck ever since she was eighteen. It wasn't unsightly and hadn't caused her any trouble. She had lived in a country district for a large part of her early life, and thought there had been one or two neighbours with goitres. Possibly there was some shortage of iodine or too much lime in the district. As Rita got older her thyroid became lumpy or nodular, as commonly happens, but she was perfectly well until she was just coming up to retirement from her job in the electricity company. Apparently without rhyme or reason, she developed what her husband put down to delayed effects of the change. She was too hot, easily got puffed, and her hair was going grey – and she wasn't her usual placid self. She went to the doctor to ask about hormone replacement therapy, and so the real problem was discovered.

Because of the age group concerned, multinodular goitre frequently leads to symptoms of strain on the heart – shortness of breath, swollen ankles and upset to the rhythm of the heart. This last may develop into the rapid irregularity called atrial fibrillation (see Chapter 8). Any of the other symptoms of overactive thyroid can, of course, also arise.

Tests

Blood tests in this type show an increase in thyroid hormone, but not as much as in Graves'. A scintigram (see page 122) shows some lumpy areas working flat out, others doing nothing. An electrical tracing of the heart's action – an electrocardiogram – may be done to provide exact information (see Chapter 11).

How to get well

The same treatments are available as for Graves' disease (page 48):

- *Beta-blockers* alone are not enough, but they take the edge off the discomfort for a start.
- *Antithyroid drugs* are ineffective – relapse is inevitable.
- *Radioiodine* would probably be your choice, unless your goitre is big, ugly or awkward, when surgery would be preferred. In this disorder a second dose is required in 25 per cent of patients, but, on the credit side, there is less likelihood of your switching right over into thyroid deficiency.

Special care, if necessary, for your heart and circulatory problems is dealt with in Chapter 8.

Toxic nodule

A solitary 'hot spot' is ten times more likely in a woman than in a man, and is usually found in the over-forty age range. The nodule may have been present for a long time, as with multinodular goitre, but a single lump, whether overactive or not, is more likely to be noticeable. A large nodule is more likely to become overactive than a smaller one, and a hot nodule is often about 1 to 1¼ inches across. The rest of the gland shrinks and produces nothing if one part is making too much hormone: this reduces the severity of the symptoms, by comparison with Graves' or multinodular overactive thyroid.

Tests

- *Blood tests* for hormones usually show an increase in T_4 and T_3, but occasionally in T_3 only.
- *Scintigram* (page 122) This pinpoints a hot nodule dramatically as a rule, but in 5 to 10 per cent the overactive part doesn't show up.

- *Fine-needle aspiration* (page 123)   This is the definitive test. A very fine needle is used to obtain a minute sample of the tissue of the nodule. You hardly feel anything. The advantage of this test is precise information and the certain elimination of any possibility of the lump's being cancerous.

How to get well

As with toxic multinodular goitre, beta-blockers are only useful temporarily, and the antithyroid drugs don't work properly (see pages 48 and 52).

- *Radioiodine* (see page 129)   will knock out the overactive nodule, and the rest of the thyroid will gradually recover and resume normal production.
- *Surgery* (see page 131)   will be your choice if the lump is unsightly or gets in the way, or if for some reason your doctor thinks there is a risk that it could become cancerous. There is some evidence that having had X-rays of the neck early in life may make the gland more susceptible to cancer.

Hashitoxicosis

In a minority of people in the early stages of Hashimoto's disease (see page 35), some of the symptoms of thyroid *over*activity flare up for a few weeks. These may be the first indication you get of anything wrong, or you may merely be aware of a small goitre, of rubbery consistency. You start feeling ill, losing weight and suffering from looseness of the bowels. You are aware of palpitations, and feeling the heat.

Tests

The give-away is the presence of antithyroid antibodies in your blood. Later in Hashimoto's disease, the level of these antibodies sinks to an undetectable level.

Treatment

This is best kept simple, since it will probably not be needed for more than two months maximum. Beta-blockers will help you through this period.

De Quervain's thyroiditis

This painful goitre has an early stage of overactivity of the gland, leading to the characteristic symptoms (see page 24). This stage may last for several months and calls for the use of beta-blockers in addition to the treatment for the inflammation (see page 128).

Excess of iodine

It must have seemed like a wonderful breakthrough when, in the nineteenth century, it was discovered that lack of iodine was the cause of the goitres, myxoedema and cretinism common in many areas at that time. Doctors and public-health officers enthusiastically added iodine to flour, table salt and water. A lot of people were made really ill by overdosing with iodine – notably in Switzerland, a mountainous country with a reputation for goitre.

In some people the reaction of their thyroid to all this iodine was underactivity. Others, more dangerously, were precipitated into toxic overactivity. Nowadays such mistakes over quantity cannot occur, and it is unusual for anyone to become ill from an excess, although there was a recent outbreak in Tasmania – an iodine-containing disinfectant had been used to clean milking utensils.

You are more likely to have a toxic reaction if you already have a goitre, or if you live in an area where the normal diet is low in iodine – for instance in Tuscany or parts of Germany.

Current sources of extra iodine

(a) *Radiographic contrast media* Chemicals used in special X-ray investigations, often of the kidneys or gall bladder.

(b) *Iodine tincture or powder* used to disinfect extensive wounds or burns.

In both (a) and (b) any toxic effects are delayed until several weeks later, because the gland takes time to convert the excess iodine into excess hormone.

(c) *Kelp* This is a seaweed available in health-food shops in various forms. Taken to excess it provides too much iodine for the thyroid to cope with.

(d) *Potassium iodide* This is an ingredient in some cough mixtures, which could cause trouble if taken over a long period.

(e) *Betadine* is used in mouthwashes, and too much may be absorbed.

With (a) to (e) the offending chemical can be discontinued or not repeated. While the excess iodine is still being processed by the thyroid you may have such symptoms as palpitations and overheating, but a beta-blocker (see page 128) will tide you over this limited period.

(f) *Amiodarone* This medicine can be more of a problem. It is an excellent regularizer for disorders of the rhythm of the heart, and usually needs to be taken indefinitely. The daily dose provides 100 times as much iodine as a normal diet. In most cases the symptoms of overproduction of thyroid hormone don't appear until you have been on the drug for about thirty months – or it can be as long as three years. Then they come suddenly.

Men are more likely to be affected than women, and they are likely to be restless and trembly, and perhaps develop a small goitre. The original heart problems may worsen.

It may not be safe to stop the drug, and anyway it remains in the system for about a month after the last dose. Beta-blockers and antithyroid drugs are usually given, but the latter take a particularly long time to have an effect. Radioiodine is useless, since the thyroid is already as full as it can be of ordinary iodine. Sometimes operation is the only possible treatment, if the amiodarone must be continued.

Excess of thyroid hormone by mouth

There are three reasons for this situation:

(a) Misjudgement of the dose, usually through failing to arrange regular blood tests, when you are on T_4 for underactive thyroid.
(b) A vain attempt to cure 'metabolic insufficiency', in the belief that it must be due to lack of thyroid – see page 40.
(c) The mistaken use of thyroxine to reduce weight.

Charlotte weighed fifteen stone and looked fat. She was fifty and fed up with it. She pressurized two separate doctors to prescribe T_4 and took double doses, hoping to speed up her metabolism and 'burn off' the unwanted fat. Her appetite increased, and when she had her minor heart attack, her weight was sixteen stone.

Thyroid hormones are useless as a slimming aid, because taking the extra switches off your own thyroid production. It can be harmful to your heart and blood pressure.

All you need do, in (a) to (c), is cut out or reduce the thyroid by mouth, and monitor the blood level for as long as your doctor advises.

Disorders of the pituitary gland

This gland in the brain produces TSH – thyroid-stimulating hormone. In the rare event of a pituitary tumour, it may make too much TSH and overstimulate the thyroid. Treatment is concentrated on the pituitary.

Cancer

Cancer of the thyroid is uncommon (see page 25), and it is extremely rare for it to cause thyrotoxicosis. Either a large dose of radioiodine or surgery would be the best treatment (see page 129).

Rarely a tumour of the testis or of the ovary may lead to symptoms of overactive thyroid. As with pituitary tumour, the most important treatment is for the underlying disorder, but a beta-blocker (see page 128) may make you more comfortable in the meantime.

5

Having a baby

'Oh, my throat has come to be swollen,' so murmured the
beauty. Fearful. Quiet, my child, peace, and hearken to me:
'You have been touched by Venus's hand; softly she tells
you . . .'

J.W. Von GOETHE, The Four Seasons, 1790

Having a baby – it's the essence of being alive, the most funda-
mental experience of all. No one who wants it should miss it. Your
thyroid plays a key role from before conception to after the birth.

Take Rob and Vicky. They'd DIYed their flat to perfection and
paid the last instalment on the Micra. Vicky stopped the pill and
started window-shopping in Mothercare. After six months:
nothing. Vicky's mother and the doctor both said it was early
days, so they went on trying. They'd always had a good sex life,
but now Vicky found she couldn't summon up any enthusiasm.
Her periods were a nuisance, too – heavier than before, and
irregular. She blamed them for feeling washed out.
    A thyroid test showed that Vicky had an underactive thyroid.
She was prescribed thyroxine tablets, and three months later she
became pregnant.

Fertility

For an intending parent of either sex, a normally working thyroid
gland is essential.

Underactive thyroid

Man's side   There is an abysmal lack of sexual interest, a low sperm
count and, at the worst, impotence. This not a life sentence: normal
feelings, function and fertility are rapidly restored with thyroxine
treatment.

Woman's angle   As with Vicky, an underactive thyroid means loss
of libido, plus menorrhagia – heavy periods – with an underlying
failure to ovulate. Sometimes the periods stop, and the woman's
hopes are raised that she is pregnant. Treatment is effective.

The symptoms of an underactive thyroid come on so gradually, and seem so unimportant at first – slowing down a little, mild weight gain, constipation – that it's not surprising they are often overlooked. Sometimes it is only because of investigations for infertility that the true problem shows up.

Overactive thyroid

Man's side Fertility is certainly reduced, but sexual interest and performance may remain normal or fall off. In some men a swelling of the breast area occurs, and a few are impotent.

Woman's angle Periods are infrequent and scanty, and may peter out. Even before this, the monthly release of an egg for possible fertilization – ovulation – is in abeyance, so conception is unlikely. If you do become pregnant, there is high risk of miscarriage. An overactive thyroid is harder to ignore than an underactive one and treatment is necessary for health and comfort, since the anxiety, restlessness and palpitations interfere with normal living.

If infertility is due to either an underactive or an overactive thyroid, treatment of the thyroid fault automatically corrects the infertility. The one proviso is that, for a woman with an overactive gland, special precautions over the type of treatment are needed if pregnancy is in prospect. See pages 62–3 for details.

How your thyroid functions during pregnancy

The thyroid is a vital ally in the whole project of being pregnant. It enables your body to function as usual for ten months, while providing for the total support of a new human being inside you. It stimulates and directs the baby's all-over growth throughout, with particular relevance to his or her mental development in the last six months.

What you notice

You may feel off colour for the first few weeks while your system adjusts, but after that, thanks to your thyroid, it is 90 per cent positive:

- You don't feel the cold, although you may not appreciate the heat so much towards the end.
- Your circulation is better than usual.
- You look well.
- You have a good, but not excessive, appetite, and a good digestion to go with it.

- You put on weight, but this time you don't have to cut down on your favourite foods.
- Your mood shifts gradually towards greater optimism.
- If you have any autoimmune problems – for instance rheumatoid arthritis – they improve.
- Your thyroid gland – working hard – may get a little bigger and feel warm to the touch.

The essential factor is your metabolism – the rate at which you burn up your food. By the last few months it will be running at 15 per cent above normal. Your heart beats faster and more strongly, and, because you are using more oxygen, your breathing is quicker and deeper. There is more blood in circulation, with a generous flow through the womb – and the thyroid. In fact the output from the heart is up by 30 to 40 per cent by the twenty-seventh week of pregnancy, though after that it settles down to a slower, steady rate until the birth. These last weeks are important for the subtle and far-reaching developments taking place in the baby's nervous system and brain.

You will be eating a little more, but the increase doesn't amount to 'eating for two'. Your body's improved efficiency easily provides for body-building – the baby's and yours. He or she goes up from 0 to 6½ lbs and your weight may climb by as much as 17 lb. A large proportion of this is fluid: the baby's water cushion of amniotic fluid, your extra blood, and an increase in body water. In addition there is development of the breasts (about 2 lbs), the womb itself and the placenta, through which the baby receives his or her supplies. There is also a small fat reserve, to allow for breast-feeding later.

As well as all this construction work – and thyroid hormones are vital in making new protein – your metabolism has to provide you with extra energy. Your muscles have a heavier load to carry, and there is a bigger body to nourish and keep going.

During the first twelve weeks the foetus has no thyroid gland and is entirely dependent on you for his or her thyroid hormone. After that he or she produces most of the necessary supply, but needs a 20 per cent top-up from you.

Thyroid tests

These reflect all this special activity. A straight T_4 estimation shows an increase, but this is deceptive – the concentration of free, ready-to-use T_4 and T_3 is only marginally increased, within the normal range; the difference is in the 'bound' form. Before it is released to do its work, locally, thyroxine is attached to a particular protein, which carries it round in the circulation for when it is needed somewhere. It is rather like a milk float taking pintas round the streets and dropping off supplies where they are wanted.

Nourishment

During the first three months of pregnancy your body can supply most of what the foetus needs without strain. In the later months your intake of food may fall short of requirements – not in bulk, but for instance in calcium and various vitamins. Supplements are usually necessary.

With all the metabolic activity going on, it is hardly surprising that the thyroid – a major controller, and very busy – should get bigger, like a well-exercised muscle. It may not be only the extra demands on the thyroid that make it work so hard: it may also be struggling to make the best of a relative shortage of its raw material, iodine. You may live in an area where the ordinary diet provides quite sufficient iodine for you, but not for anything extra like pregnancy. It is significant that in Scotland 80 per cent of mothers-to-be develop a pregnancy goitre, while in the USA, where the dietary intake of iodine is four times greater, this is a rarity. An added drain on iodine supplies during pregnancy is an increased iodine loss in the urine, due to the kidneys being more active than usual.

If your normal diet is near the borderline of a satisfactory iodine content, as in many parts of Europe, it is wise to make sure of an adequate amount from the beginning of pregnancy. This is a very small quantity, easily provided by having sea fish once or twice a week (sardines, for example, which are also an excellent source of iron and calcium), or by using sea salt for cooking and the table. An overload of iodine is definitely harmful to the foetus, so don't be too enthusiastic, however.

All we have discussed in the last couple of pages is what happens during pregnancy when the thyroid is functioning absolutely perfectly. Special care is needed if your thyroid is underactive, overactive or enlarged.

Goitre

If you have a simple goitre, without any symptoms of over- or underactivity, you should have a thyroid test – if possible including an antibody screen. If your T_4 and T_3 levels are normal but the presence of antithyroid antibodies in your blood indicates an autoimmune process going on quietly (Hashimoto's disorder – see page 35), you need take no action apart from having thyroid checks once or twice during the pregnancy and – most importantly – afterwards.

Immunity reactions, including the Hashimoto type, all subside during pregnancy, so that you don't react against the baby – an invader in your body who is 50 per cent different from you.

Underactive thyroid

If this is shown by the tests, whether or not you have the slow-down symptoms, it is essential to start thyroxine treatment straightaway. In this case, or if you are already on T_4 for Hashimoto's disease, it is important to keep to the same dose throughout the pregnancy. This must be regardless of the simple T_4 tests – these will show an increase, but not in the free thyroxine, which is what matters (see page 119). If you feel hot, and your pulse is fast and strong, don't assume this means that you are taking too much of the hormone – pregnancy itself leads to these effects. Check with your doctor. One of the thyroid tests – that for TSH (thyroid-stimulating hormone) – will tell him if you need an increase in the dosage. Your baby's development depends upon a sufficient supply of thyroid hormone (see Chapter 6).

The birth A tendency to underactive thyroid will give you problems with this.

Overactive thyroid

It is unusual to conceive if you have an unrecognized overactive thyroid, but no surprise if you have had treatment for it. Ideally, if you know in advance that you are hyperthyroid and want to plan ahead, you will get the thyroid problem sorted out permanently before starting a family.

A lasting cure means radioiodine or an operation. Most people, given a free choice, would prefer the medication to surgery, but there has to be a four- or five-month gap between taking the radioactive material and conception. After that, there is no risk to the baby's normal development. If your plans don't allow for this delay, then an operation to remove seven-eighths of the gland is a once-and-for-all option. Otherwise, you can with care use one of the antithyroid drugs – carbimazole, methimazole or propylthiour-acil – to control the thyroid problem while you are trying for a baby.

Overactive thyroid

During pregnancy If you have the common autoimmune type of overactive thyroid, your symptoms and test results will improve slightly because of the effect of pregnancy on the immune system. You will probably still need treatment – at any rate in the early stages.

Another possibility is that you develop Graves' disease for the first time when you are already pregnant. This can be difficult to recognize, because many of the indications of overactive thyroid also crop up in pregnancy. They include feeling hot and sweaty, passing water extra frequently, a strong heartbeat and some anxiety. Blood tests and a pulse rate that stays obstinately above ninety beats per minute plus failure to put on weight as you should show that your symptoms are due to illness.

Whether the overactive thyroid is a new development or already established, you must have treatment, for your own health and comfort and to lessen the risk of miscarriage, especially in the first few months. Unfortunately the antithyroid drugs pass through the placenta and reach the foetus. Too much could damage his thyroid. This means that you must keep to the smallest dose compatible with your feeling well. The usual choice in the United States is propylthiouracil, which is also the least harmful during breast-feeding. In Europe carbimazole is favoured during the pregnancy, with propylthiouracil after the birth.

Either way, no antithyroid drugs should be taken during the last four to six weeks before the expected birth day. This is the time of maximum brain development for the baby, and it is important that his own thyroid is not pushed into underactivity by his mother's antithyroid medicine. The only exception is if the doctor has some reason to think that the baby is at risk of being born with an overactive thyroid himself. There is a blood test which is not available in all districts, for a specific antithyroid antibody, TRAb, which sets off Graves' disease. If you have this in your blood, there is a small chance – 1 in 70 – of the baby's thyroid being affected. In this situation, if there are other indications, for instance in the foetal heart rate, it may be considered best for you to take antithyroid medication throughout (see Chapter 6).

It is more likely that your doctor will be aiming at keeping the antithyroid medication to a minimum. Regular testing will help to establish the dosage you need, or adding a beta-blocker (see pages 128–9) if you have unpleasant symptoms of overactivity. This will not affect the baby.

Often iodine is used to switch an overactive thyroid down

quickly, but you cannot have this during pregnancy, nor any other iodine-containing medicine or wound disinfectant. Iodine can cause a large goitre to develop in the foetus, if he receives a substantial dose through his mother. Radioiodine treatment is out, of course, but an operation is a possibility if the overactive thyroid is causing the mother distress. The middle three months of pregnancy are the safest time for this, with the least danger of bringing on a miscarriage. The taking of iodine to quieten down the gland in the run-up to surgery on the thyroid (see page 50) is risky to the foetus, but a combination of antithyroid medication and a beta-blocker can be used instead. Operating without settling the thyroid first can be dangerous.

Thyroid storm This is overactivity of a thyroid that has run out of control. It is very rare, but an emergency when it occurs. It requires instant hospitalization and energetic antithyroid measures. These are life-saving and take priority over everything else.

Eclampsia – a complication of late pregnancy, involving raised blood pressure – plus the birth itself can precipitate a thyroid storm if the mother's overactive thyroid has not been treated effectively. The way to prevent any risk is to keep all your antenatal appointments meticulously and make sure you have regular thyroid tests.

The birth

Apart from the exceptional rarity of thyroid storm, giving birth will not be affected by an overactive thyroid. At this time the common autoimmune type of overactive thyroid is usually in abeyance, to return later.

After the birth (post-partum)

Testing the baby's thyroid

However normal your thyroid and the pregnancy, and however beautiful your baby, it is important for him or her to have a blood test at five to seven days old. This is to pick up the 1 in 3,000 chance of thyroid deficiency. Even at this rate, it is six times as likely as PKU (phenylketonuria), the other rare congenital disorder that can seriously hold back mental development if it is not spotted early. Your baby may have extra tests if you have had any thyroid problems (see Chapter 6).

Looking after you

It is natural and understandable to feel exhausted but excited after the exertion of giving birth or the drama of a Caesarean. The well-known 'after-baby blues' affects many mothers to some extent in the first week or two. It amounts to a few days' weepiness, although underneath you know there is everything to be happy about. In the ordinary course, your thyroxine output dips briefly after the birth, but the effect isn't noticeable.

Ordinarily your physical and emotional strength pick up during the first month, but there's a 1 in 6 chance of developing a thyroid problem in three to six months. This is usually temporary.

Post-partum hypothyroidism You can suspect that your thyroid has slipped into underactivity if you become tired, weak and depressed after you should have got over the initial reaction to having a baby. You find you can't concentrate, and your memory is dodgy. You haven't much appetite, but your weight seems to be stuck where it was when you had the baby, instead of reverting to your pre-pregnancy state. This is not a severe case of the blues, or a matter of being neurotic, but a real chemical deficiency of thyroid hormones. Testing will show this.

It is usually worthwhile to have a short course of hormone replacement. In three-quarters of mothers the problem is short-lived, lasting only a few months. That leaves a quarter who continue to run low in thyroid indefinitely. This is all the more likely if you have a goitre, had been hypothyroid previously, or just have antithyroid antibodies according to the tests. If you were on thyroxine tablets before and during the pregnancy, you will certainly need to continue with them, since the beneficial effects on your immune system stop with the birth.

In any case, you should continue taking the medication as long as tests indicate that you need it. At the proper dosage, the tablets have no side-effects and do not affect the baby if you breast-feed.

Post-partum thyroiditis This arises more often than underactivity after a birth, particularly in North America and Japan. It is an autoimmune problem, but not due to the same antibodies as Graves' disease. It is also called 'silent thyroiditis' because, although there is inflammation of the gland, it isn't painful or tender, unlike in de Quervain's thyroiditis (see page 24).

You develop the tremor, palpitations and sharp loss of weight and general restless anxiety that are characteristic of an overactive thyroid. You feel hot and tired, and, just at this time when you need all the sleep you can get, you sleep badly. Probably your thyroid will be its normal size, but if it is at all swollen this will be only slightly. This condition can ruin the delight of having a new baby, but sadly it is often dismissed by doctors and husbands as natural worrying and inability to cope – especially if you are a first-time mother.

This phase, untreated, lasts two to four months. After that you may shift gear into reverse – a stage of underactivity, with slow-down, depression, constipation and fatigue. This state of affairs can last for weeks, months or indefinitely, or hardly develop at all. A goitre appears in nearly half of all those who suffer post-partum thyroiditis.

What to do If the symptoms of overactivity are mild, it may be possible to control them with a beta-blocker which has no ill-effect on breast-feeding. More likely you will need an antithyroid, and propylthiouracil is the least liable to get through into your milk in harmful amounts. One proviso: if your doctor wants you to have a scintigram to help confirm the diagnosis (see page 122), you must stop breast-feeding for four days afterwards, otherwise the radioactive iodine which is used for this special X-ray might harm the baby. It is washed out of your system well before four days.

If you are not breast-feeding, all options are open, including a course of a steroid medicine to cut the thyroiditis short.

Future outlook With either underactive thyroid or post-partum thyroiditis there is a good chance that the disorder will last only weeks or a few months before you are back to normal. On the other hand, if you have had post-partum thyroiditis once, you are likely to have it again when you have another child. Post-partum hypo-thyroidism may also recur on subsequent occasions, but the chances are somewhat less.

6

Babies before and after birth

Baby-in-the-making

From the moment of conception, when sperm meets ovum and the miracle begins, your baby depends on you, the mother, for warmth, protection, nourishment and a supply of hormones. The thyroid hormones, T_4 and T_3, have a vital role to play right through pregnancy and beyond. They work hand-in-hand with growth hormone for the baby's general development – including the development of such important organs as the lungs, heart and liver – but in two areas their influence is dominant:

- *the brain and the nervous system*, particularly the cerebral cortex, where ideas come from and thinking goes on, and the cerebellum, which controls the coordination of muscle movement;
- *the bone system*, which involves height, facial features, and shape, and the skull – the strong box that contains the brain.

In the first few weeks the foetus is almost microscopic in size, but after that there is a measurable change every week. At twelve weeks, he or she will be about 4 inches long, at twenty weeks 8 inches and at forty weeks a little over 20 inches, depending on a normal thyroid input.

To start off with the embryo absorbs all she needs directly from the tissues of the womb, where she is nestling. Everything you carry in your bloodstream, including the requisite thyroid hormones, simply soaks into the embryo, all over. This arrangement works satisfactorily while the embryo is only a minute bundle of cells, but is inadequate by ten or eleven weeks. The baby-in-the-making then needs a more efficient method. Urgently, your womb grows, and a part is adapted to make the placenta. This acts as Harrods to the baby's requirements, with an exclusive transport system along the umbilical cord. The placenta also acts as a kind of doorman, preventing certain substances from getting through. Although thyroid hormones are absolutely essential for foetal development, they are on the exclusion list.

Progress does not come to a halt. While the placenta has been evolving as a supply service, the baby has been busy forming her own thyroid gland. This starts as a lump near the back of her tongue at about the third week. From there, over the ensuing weeks, the newly grown gland gradually shifts its position, moving under the jaw and into the neck, into the prearranged slot. It divides into two lobes, one each side of the voice-box, joined by a narrow strip of tissue. This complicated process goes astray surprisingly seldom (see below).

When the foetus is about six weeks old, the developing thyroid learns to trap iodine, and then to use it to make T_4 and T_3. By the time the foetus has to rely on the placenta for supplies from you, her own thyroid is capable of producing enough hormone for her needs. A small percentage still gets through from your blood, but in general, from twelve weeks onwards it hardly affects the baby if you are hypothyroid. The baby's thyroid output increases steadily as she grows – and how she grows! It takes twenty-two weeks to achieve a weight of 1 lb. This is trebled to 3 lb by the thirty-second week, reaches 4½ lb at the thirty-sixth, and a final weight of about 7 lb is achieved at forty weeks.

Building at this rate demands a high-speed metabolism – twice the rate of an adult. This is reflected in the increasing heart rate. The foetal heart can just be detected at four weeks, running at sixty-five beats a minute, much the same as in us adults, but by the end of pregnancy the rate is more than double: 140 per minute. For your heart to go that fast you would have to run until you were puffed. The thyroid is in charge of both metabolism and heart rate.

During the final two months of life in the womb there is a concentration on brain development, including the 'governing' parts – the pituitary and the hypothalamus. These provide information and instructions to all areas of the nervous and hormonal systems, including the thyroid. At this stage and continuing through the baby's first eighteen months in the outside world, there is a massive increase in the number of brain cells. These are precious, since they cannot be produced or replaced later: they form the stock of mental material for the whole of the baby's life. A steady, sufficient flow of thyroxine is essential for this far-reaching development. No amount of money, medicine or education can make up for a deficit of thyroid hormone before birth.

At the same time other organs, necessary for life, such as lungs and liver, are continuing their development. These are not fully mature and may not work very well when the baby is born, especially if she is premature. This does not apply to the thyroid, unless the baby arrives extremely early, since the gland has an important and at times life-saving role immediately after the birth.

Birth

The baby leaves the warmth and security of the womb and her supply line – the umbilical cord – is cut. The shock of the cold makes her gasp – and breathe. It also stimulates the thyroid to pour out a huge amount of T_4, and, the moment the cord is cut, T_3 is also released in quantity. Although the baby's temperature plummets initially, by the time she is seven hours old it is up to normal. This is because her metabolic rate, burning up fuel, has shot up by nearly 30 per cent under the influence of the extra thyroid hormones. This peaks around the second day, running at double the adult rate. The thyroid of a very premature infant, younger than thirty-five weeks, cannot react so vigorously, which is one of the reasons why tiny premature babies have to start their lives in an incubator.

The hormone levels sink gradually over a few weeks, but remain higher than the adult level during the first four or five years of especially rapid growth.

In her first few days, before feeding is established, the baby has to depend on her own reserves for fuel. This is in part responsible for the normal weight loss in the first week.

The above is the everyday wonder that we take for granted, but nature isn't a production line. There are individual variations, most of them irrelevant but a few that you need to watch out for, so as to ward off later trouble for your child.

Screening tests for deficiency of thyroid and for phenylketonuria are carried out after the fifth day, when the dramatic fluctuations in thyroid activity have settled down. The method is to prick the baby's heel for a drop of blood: at this age the skin is as thin and soft in that area as anywhere.

Screening is useful for picking out the majority of clear cases of lack of thyroid, but no test is 100 per cent accurate. Personal observation is the safety-net, necessary for someone as precious as your baby, on the threshold of life.

Shortage of thyroid

It is because of the disastrous effects of uncorrected lack of thyroid hormones that governments all over the world have set up screening programmes for the newborn. Although there are 2,999 babies with a normal thyroid to one with a deficiency, it is cost-effective to the state to pick up that one, who would need special care all his life without treatment. The point is that treatment is simple, cheap and effective – so long as it is started within weeks of birth. From a mother's point of view, it saves her child's beauty, brains and happiness for the rest of his life. A baby's thyroid deficiency may stem from a number of sources:

- Some risks to the baby's thyroid come through his or her mother, and can often be avoided.
- Some thyroid deficiencies result from minor manufacturing faults in the baby which are not life-threatening but must be dealt with for full health.

Through the parents

Either parent may pass on genes which increase the chances of a thyroid disorder, or an autoimmune tendency in general, but the mother is more intimately concerned, particularly if she has had a thyroid problem at any time. The following are the most likely problem areas:

Recent radioiodine treatment for overactive thyroid would imply a major mistake and/or a failure of contraception. Because the delicate foetal thyroid would be destroyed and because of the danger of general radiation effects, if you were unlucky enough to be in this situation you would probably give serious consideration to termination of pregnancy. You could start again six months from the date of taking the radioiodine.

Antithyroid medicines – carbimazole, methimazole and propylthiouracil – given to you for an overactive thyroid, pass through the placenta and can affect the baby's thyroid. Your dosage needs careful monitoring, keeping it as low as possible while yet controlling your hormone level. The antithyroid should be suspended in the last four to six weeks of pregnancy, and a beta-blocker such as propanolol used to keep you comfortable, if necessary.

Antithyroid antibodies If you have had the autoimmune condition Hashimoto's disease at any time and you still carry a substantial amount of the antithyroid antibody in your blood, there is a small risk that the unwanted antibody will directly affect the baby's thyroid.

If you are currently on treatment for underactive thyroid from any cause, including Hashimoto, and you are pregnant, discuss with your doctor whether you should now increase your thyroxine medication slightly. In no circumstance should you reduce or stop it, even if you feel well and your thyroxine level is up (see page 61).

It is important to have your thyroid checked out regularly throughout the pregnancy if you have ever had any thyroid disorder.

Medicines or foods that you might take can upset the baby's thyroid. Apart from a once-off dose of contrast material for an X-ray of your upper digestive system (unlikely anyway while you are pregnant), no harm to the baby will result unless you take the possibly offending substance consistently for some time. Medicines that matter are those containing iodides, such as some cough mixtures, and amiodarone for the heart; lithium, for mood illnesses; antipyrine for asthma; sulphonamides for infections; and some antidiabetic drugs. Discuss with your doctor if you are on any of these.

On the food front, avoid an excess of the sprout and cabbage family of vegetables; soya; sweet corn; almonds, and the health food kelp.

Even if you are not taking a medicine or eating much of a food that could interfere with the baby's thyroid, you may live in an area where there is a general shortage of iodine in the soil and water and thus in your diet and you may not be passing on enough iodine for his needs. This is certainly the case in Zaïre, and in many parts of India, where there is also genetic thyroid weakness, and in pockets all over the Third World. All that is needed is for you to ensure a reasonable intake of iodine for yourself during the pregnancy, but not an excess (see page 60).

Faults in the baby's development

The transformation from a single cell to 6½ lb or so of living, breathing, crying humanity is a remarkable achievement. Even the development of the thyroid gland itself is a complicated affair. It is no wonder that sometimes – amazingly seldom – some details don't go according to plan. We don't know the reasons for the following problems that do occasionally arise.

Agenesis This means that the development of the thyroid has never got past the bud stage, and it can hardly produce any hormone.

Dysgenesis This is one step better than agenesis, but development is incomplete. The gland may not have got as far as forming two lobes.

Agenesis and dysgenesis between them account for 80 to 90 per cent of babies born with a lack of thyroid hormone. Girls are affected twice as often as boys.

Dyshormonogenesis This is extremely rare. The baby's thyroid looks normal enough, but either it doesn't respond to the thyroid-stimulating hormone from the pituitary, or it hasn't developed the knack of synthesizing its own T_4 and T_3. They are complicated chemically, and it took the world's chemists until 1914 to produce a single crystal of thyroxine, and another quarter century for triiodothyronine, T_3.

Ectopic thyroid This term means that the gland is in the wrong place, having never completed the journey from the tongue to the front of the neck (see page 67) or having overshot the mark and landed up behind the breastbone. Most likely it never got started, but has developed as a reddish-purple lump on the tongue – a so-called *lingual thyroid*. If for any reason it becomes swollen it can be a great nuisance in this situation, getting in the way of swallowing, crying and even breathing. It may cause similar problems behind the breastbone, but usually much later (see page 18). If the gland stops short of its proper destination, it may appear as a lump in the midline of the neck.

With any of these developmental mistakes the thyroid is unlikely to work perfectly. The baby may be born already hypothyroid, or the shortfall in hormones may not become obvious until later (see page 78).

What you may notice

Before birth Since most thyroid-deficient babies seem perfectly normal when they are born, there isn't much likelihood that there will be anything obviously wrong before then. For one thing, in the womb, she could probably get by on the small amount of hormone leaking through the placenta. A thyroid-deficient baby is likely to be especially peaceful, with none of that energetic kicking that mothers-to-be complain about. On the other hand, most babies settle for a quiet life towards the end of pregnancy: they simply haven't got room to move. An X-ray would show that the hypothyroid baby's bone development is delayed, and the last pre-birth indication is that she stays on well after the expected birth date – more than two weeks. Your doctor won't let this go on.

If there's a suspicion that the baby is lacking in thyroid, taking extra yourself doesn't help in the later months of pregnancy – the

71

placenta won't let it get through. Occasionally it has been thought worthwhile to inject thyroxine into the amniotic fluid surrounding the foetus, but generally it is enough to check the situation when the baby arrives and start replacement treatment as soon as it becomes clear that it is needed.

After the birth   Usually a hypothyroid baby looks perfect when he first emerges. His muscles may look slightly bigger than most babies', and to the doctor the fontanelle – the gap in the head bones where they haven't finally joined together – may seem a little large. The screening test is positive if either the T_4 level is low or the TSH (thyroid-stimulating hormone) is high, depending on the test employed. It means that the baby needs a thyroid supplement, whatever the underlying cause of the shortage. This can be started at a fortnight old and must be begun by the time he is two months.

If he, or more likely she, has been deprived for some time before birth, although he may be of average length and weight, his bones will show immaturity on an X-ray. His brain will also show underdevelopment and slow electrical waves if he is given an EEG (electroencephalogram), a recording of its activity, picked up through the scalp.

Without any treatment, nothing obvious may happen for several years, but all the time irreversible damage will be affecting the baby's brain. Early signs of too little thyroid hormone are often difficult to recognize, and you should not blame yourself if you fail to notice them. The baby sleeps a lot, isn't much interested in feeding, is slow to put on weight, and just doesn't make progress. She doesn't get in a temper and kick and scream – ever – and she's constipated. She may have a rather bulging tummy and perhaps an umbilical hernia, a small protuberance at the navel.

In about a third of thyroid-deprived babies there may be one or more of these symptoms:

- breathing difficulties or noisy breathing;
- a hoarse cry;
- a low temperature: 36°C or less;
- prolonged baby jaundice;
- a big tongue;
- floppy muscles.

Whatever the situation at the beginning, later on the baby will be slow to reach the milestones for smiling, talking and getting teeth, and later still she will be clumsy and poorly coordinated for skilled movements. None of this need happen, nor the terrible mental retardation that could wreck her, or his, life. All that is needed is to start treatment by the time she is six weeks old. Even without a positive screening test, hints of thyroid lack, such as those above, should not be ignored.

Transient hypothyroidism

It is not uncommon, especially if the baby was premature, for it to take several weeks for a new baby's thyroid to start producing enough thyroxine for his needs. Another cause of a brief lack of T_4 is the use of an iodine-containing antiseptic during or after the birth. Iodine in quantity switches off the thyroid. Either way, a short course of thyroxine covers the situation, monitored by repeat tests.

Temporary hypothyroidism

This may result if the baby's thyroid has been affected by the mother's taking an antithyroid medicine during pregnancy, or if some antithyroid antibodies of the Hashimoto type have reached him from her circulation. In these cases the effect usually wears off, but T_4 is usually given for the whole of the baby's first year, and is then discontinued after a satisfactory test result.

Long-term hypothyroidism

If the baby has been born with a rudimentary thyroid gland or for some other developmental reason it cannot supply sufficient hormone, he will need to take thyroxine by mouth indefinitely. This will be by spoon, with juice or formula, at first, and later by the usual small, tasteless tablets. Babies and toddlers up to around age four have a rapid, active metabolism to help them. Weight for weight, they need a bigger dose than an adult.

Baby Christine was good – too good, as it turned out. She slept through the night right from the start, and was generally cuddly and placid – 'contented', her grandmother said. It was difficult to get her to take her feed, and Jill felt there must be something wrong with her milk. The baby was just as bored by a complementary bottle. The original screening test had been inconclusive, and a repeat two weeks later showed that Christine was mildly hypothyroid, so thyroid treatment was begun. Jill and Tim were quite unprepared for the change. Christine cried loudly and a lot, often at night. She was always hungry, and needed changing far more frequently. She was generally restless, kicking off her covers and then getting cold. The final straw was that her scanty hair all fell out. Jill told the clinic doctor.

If Christine had been having unmistakable diarrhoea and

losing weight, the doctor might have thought the dose of T_4 was too high. As it was, he merely reassured Jill that her noisy, obstreperous infant was healthy and normal. Her lost hypothyroid hair would soon be replaced by much better silky-soft hair. Incidentally, the doctor told Jill that her breast-feeding was helpful, providing Christine with a small amount of thyroid hormone as well as the other benefits.

Nothing in life is perfect if you are a parent, but T_4 treatment for hypothyroid children is excellent if it is started in early babyhood and monitored monthly through the first year. 90 per cent of babies managed in this way finish up with a normal IQ. Young Christine is now fifteen and has just landed a scholarship to one of those prestigious boys' public schools that now take a sprinkle of girls in the sixth form.

Ectopic thyroid glands may be able to produce a reasonable amount of hormone. It is usually considered best to suppress this activity (and incidentally cause the oddly-situated tissue to shrink) with iodine and antithyroid medicine, and to supply the baby with the thyroxine she needs by mouth. If the aberrant thyroid tissue doesn't shrink enough, is in the way or looks unsightly – in the middle of the neck, for instance – it can be removed surgically at a convenient time.

Thyroglossal cyst   Sometimes a small swelling in the midline of the neck turns out to be a collection of fluid in a remnant of the pathway taken by the thyroid in its developmental journey down from the tongue area. Such cysts are of no importance at this stage, but may swell up or cause other problems later, and are best removed.

Babies with too much thyroid hormone

This is one of the few circumstances involving the thyroid where the sexes are equally affected.

Before birth

Hyperthyroidism before birth is a rare occurrence, and can only happen if a mother has Graves' disease or has had it in the past and still has a high level in her blood of TRAb. This is the abnormal antibody that overstimulates the thyroid in Graves'. It passes through the placenta from mother to foetus, and the foetal thyroid is affected. The doctor would be on the alert for such an eventuality if tests showed that you had a high TRAb. He or she would be tipped off if the baby was small for dates and had a super-fast heart rate, more than 160 beats a minute, and early maturing of the bones in an X-ray. This early maturing is not a bonus, but a disadvantage that could stunt the baby's growth. In particular it is important that the bones of the skull should not join up ahead of time, since the brain has a lot of growing to do.

What to do   Whether she needs it for herself or not, the mother will probably be given an antithyroid medicine and, if she then becomes short of thyroid hormone, T_4 tablets. The neat trick is that, while the placenta will let the antithyroid through to damp down the baby's thyroid, it will keep out the thyroid hormone. Another fortunate natural arrangement is that, although the baby may have an excess of T_4 , he cannot convert it into the much more powerful T_3 until after he has left the womb.

After the birth

Too much thyroid hormone in a newborn baby is rare, and can only occur if the mother has, or has had, Graves' disease – particularly if she was unlucky enough to have marked eye problems (see page 44). Even so, the chance of the baby's being affected is only about 1 in 100. It is important to look out for the possibility, however, since it can be dangerous without prompt treatment.

If you were taking antithyroid drugs during the pregnancy, they may have a hangover effect on the baby and prevent the symptoms of excess thyroid from coming out for the first few hours or days. The indications are a low birth weight, and an irritable baby with a very fast heart rate (taken by the doctor or midwife). A child specialist is likely to be involved for such a special baby, and the specialist will probably be able to detect a slight enlargement of the baby's thyroid and will note the warm moist skin. Sometimes the baby's eyes look a little sore and puffy.

One small snag is that, now he is separated from you, the baby can convert T_4 into powerful, fast-acting T_3, so he is likely to get worse during the first few days. Tests for thyroid hormone are variable and unreliable at this stage, so the baby's appearance and behaviour are more of a give-away. If he is suffering from too much thyroid, he will lose far more than the usual post-birth fall of 5 to 10 per cent of his birth weight. Although he seems to be dissatisfied, he is likely to be a poor feeder (though some babies react the other way and are excessively hungry). He may have a fever and is obviously ill.

What to do Medicines to quieten the thyroid include an anti-thyroid, which can be given by injection to start with, iodine drops, and the beta-blocker propranolol. The baby also needs, urgently, plenty of fluids including the right chemicals ('electrolytes') to keep the blood composition correct. If he is very hot he will need cool sponging or a fan, and a sedative to help him rest. Because his metabolism is racing he will need adequate nourishment, and possibly extra oxygen. All these needs will be met, but meanwhile it is a worrying and dramatic time.

Fortunately, after a matter of a week or so, the effect of the TRAb antibody from the mother's circulation wears off and it is not replaced. In a month or two most such babies have recovered, and their parents can expect the fun and joy of having a healthy, normal baby from then on. His antithyroid medicine can gradually be withdrawn.

Graves' disease in a baby

Sometimes, disappointingly, the symptoms of overactive thyroid start coming back after a newborn baby's antithyroid medication has been withdrawn.

That's what happened with baby Mark. Felicity, his mother, was unlucky enough to develop Graves' disease, with thyroid excess, partway through the pregnancy. This settled down after a few weeks on methimazole, and she was able to stop the drug, as recommended, for the last month.

Little Mark was born rather on the small side at just under 6 lb, and it soon became clear that he had an overactive thyroid. Everyone had been alert to the possibility, so he was started on treatment right away. All went well and his weight picked up, his bowels behaved reasonably, and he slept better. Unfortunately, within a week of reducing the antithyroid the diarrhoea came back and he was fidgety and too restless to concentrate on his feeds. Obviously all this wasn't due to Felicity's antibodies, long since cleared from Mark's system. He was making his own abnormal, thyroid-stimulating antibodies, and had developed his own, independent, Graves' disease. X-ray showed his bones were maturing somewhat too fast, so it was important for them and for his brain and nervous system to get him back on effective doses of antithyroid.

Much later, when he was starting nursery school, Mark was able to give up this medication, and from then on his T_4 and T_3 ran at a normal level. Despite this he has remained a difficult child, from the point of view of his impulsive behaviour, not his physical health. If he has a further relapse, the best treatment will be radioiodine, to deal with his thyroid once and for all.

Transient thyroid overactivity

In the ordinary way a baby's system is flooded with thyroid hormones as soon as she is born and for some days afterwards. Sometimes this is enough to make her restless, sleepless and dissatisfied; she may have frequent bowel actions. She is not ill or feverish, and the whole thing evaporates within days. No treatment is needed: this is merely an exaggeration of the normal, physiological response to birth.

7

Children and adolescents

Thyroid problems are uncommon in babies but vitally important. Too little hormone can lead to irreversible long-term damage; too much can cause a life-threatening illness. In older children thyroid disorders are less of a rarity but more liable to be overlooked. It is difficult enough with an adult to recognize the onset of a thyroid problem, but at least there is a definite change in the sufferer from her usual self. Children, by nature, are changing all the time.

One of the fascinating aspects of being a parent is following how differently each child grows and develops. You don't know in advance whether he or she will be a fast or a slow developer, when his growth spurt will start or her periods begin. Einstein didn't talk until he was four, while John Stuart Mill was already reading Greek at that age. My son George was small for his age and at fifteen was set on becoming a jockey. Eighteen months later he had a tremendous growth spurt which wrecked that project. Daughters with dreams of ballet dancing sometimes run into the same problem.

There are a few physical milestones early on, but these are long past by the time the majority of thyroid disorders appear in children. All in all, it is difficult for you or even the doctor to spot straightaway a possible thyroid problem. However, your child's physical, emotional and intellectual well-being, and his or her happiness, can depend upon how discerning you are.

Underactive thyroid in childhood

Two to one the youngster affected is a girl. She is unlikely to be younger than five, while the commonest age for this problem to show up is eight. This is because even a substandard thyroid can usually muster enough hormone for a pint-size person, but an eight-year-old uses a lot of energy and is quite big. For girls this is the threshold of puberty: the breast buds normally begin their development at this age.

It is difficult to find fault with a daughter who is slipping into thyroid deficit. She is likely to be an easy child, not given to complaining, and unlikely to be falling behind at school. If a lack of thyroid doesn't come on until the child is older than two or three years, not only does treatment with T_4 ensure that her mental development will not be permanently impaired, there may be no noticeable slow-down even before the supplement is started.

Clare was seven-and-a-half when she stopped growing. It might not have been so obvious if she hadn't been a twin: Helena was unaffected. Although Clare lagged behind her sister in height, they weighed almost the same. Clare looked stocky by comparison. She had two little pads of fat just above her collar-bones, but she was not fat otherwise. Her schoolwork was up to scratch, but she didn't seem to do so well at games as before.

A thyroid test showed that she was short of T_4; and a high level of the stimulator, TSH, confirmed that Clare's thyroid wasn't keeping up with the demands on it. Because the thyroid is particularly involved with the development of bone rather than the soft tissues, the latter had been less affected when Clare's bones stopped growing. The thyroid is also essential for brain development (see page 66), but that is largely completed by the end of the toddler stage. Clare was lucky in that she didn't have even a temporary fall in intelligence.

The problem remained: why had it happened? No one in the family had a thyroid problem, nor even one of the other autoimmune disorders. The next step was a scintigram to show the position and amount of tissue that would take up iodine: thyroid in fact. Clare's scan revealed a small amount of iodine-containing tissue under her jaw. She had an ectopic thyroid – underdeveloped and in the wrong place. It was unable to provide enough hormone for Clare at this age.

Juvenile hypothyroidism

This is the medical term for Clare's problem: inadequate thyroid production in a child past babyhood but not yet pubertal. The causes include errors in development: agenesis, dysgenesis, ectopic thyroid as in Clare's case, or the rare chemical incapacity called dyshormonogenesis (see page 71). These errors are slightly more likely in a Down's syndrome youngster. Less often the hypothyroidism is the beginning of Hashimoto's disease. The mitigating factor is that the outlook with juvenile hypothyroidism is far better than when thyroid deficiency affects a baby from birth.

The possible effects of juvenile hypothyroidism are:

- swelling in the neck – not severe;
- slow-down of growth – especially in height;
- bones at an immature stage for the chronological age (seen in an X-ray);

- delayed second teeth;
- features look young for the child's age;
- being mildly overweight for height;
- small appetite;
- constipation;
- pale, sometimes yellow-tinged skin – maybe anaemia;
- disturbed sexual development – usually delayed (no body hair, small genitals, periods delayed, poor breast development). In a minority, there is the opposite effect, with sexual maturity coming on at eight or ten years;
- mental effects – generally slow, poor memory, unable to concentrate, particular problems with language.

No hypothyroid youngster will have all these problems – different children show this disorder in different ways. Clare, for instance, had no mental or psychological impairment. If, however, a child is increasingly slow, clumsy, inattentive and apparently lazy; if he doesn't remember what he's told, and into the bargain dawdles over his meals, it is easy for the parents or teacher to misinterpret the situation. Talking it through or punishment doesn't help.

What is needed   Thyroid tests regularly, and treatment with T_4, for two years initially. Because the tablets take weeks or months to make a noticeable difference the child needs a lot of support and encouragement in the meantime. He may have a difficult time at school, but it will help if the teacher is in the picture. The long-term results are excellent.

Muscular strength and coordination – what you need to play some musical instruments – are likely to remain a little below par even after treatment. Any anaemia, on the other hand, responds well. Children, weight for weight, need more hormone than adults, but the full dosage cannot be given at the start of treatment without a risk of severe psychiatric disturbance.

The main effects of the treatment are to make the child grow taller and more energetic. The latter may catch parents unprepared. Sometimes there is too big a build-up of thyroid hormones and the youngster becomes hyperactive and distractible, and may begin doing badly at school. In these circumstances the thyroid test will distinguish between successful, normal recovery and the need to cut down the medication.

The twins are both at college now, but Clare is still 1½ inches shorter than Helena and her periods started later.

Early childhood hypothyroidism

This is not the same as juvenile hypothyroidism, and not as common. It is based on a congenital lack of thyroid, but if the shortfall is incomplete it may take over a year before there are definite indications:

- sluggishness, including the bowels;
- missing developmental milestones, slow to talk:
- slow growth;
- coarse, scanty hair;
- the head seems extra large, the face becoming broader and flatter;
- teeth are slow to come through.

Tests are urgent, with thyroid treatment to follow (see page 124).

Look-alike problems

Pauline's mother, Esmé, was certain in her own mind that her ten-year-old was suffering from lack of thyroid. Like Esmé herself, she was overweight, rather a slow child, always behind-hand, and not keeping up at school. She just didn't seem to be interested, and she also skived out of games whenever she could. The family doctor arranged thyroid tests – all negative – but allowed himself to be persuaded into trying the effect of a short course of thyroxine. Apart from an increase in an already healthy appetite, the result was zilch.

The truth of the matter was that young Pauline was depressed: she was called 'Piggy' at school and got humiliatingly out of breath at sport. When she and Esmé together switched to a healthier diet, Pauline got in better shape. Her energy, concentration and mood improved.

It is always comforting to believe that anything that goes wrong is due to 'glands' and isn't anybody's fault (see page 40). It is prudent to have a thyroid test if there is any suspicion of a problem, but if the result is negative it can only do harm to take hormone tablets. Some of the reasons why parents may suspect a thyroid disorder but be proved wrong include:

- acne;
- delayed puberty;
- being overweight;
- lagging behind at school;
- constipation;

- being physically inactive;
- a passive attitude, lack of assertiveness (especially in a boy).

These characteristics could figure in a hypothyroid disorder, but equally they may merely be aspects of individual variation, plus possibly, as in Pauline's case, depression. The laboratory tests are the best guide.

Overactive thyroid in childhood

This is, as usual, more prevalent in girls – increasingly so as they grow older and produce more oestrogen, the female sex hormone. When boys do have this disorder, they tend to suffer more severely, however.

It is rare for a child to have an overactive thyroid before the age of five; the usual age of onset is around ten. There is a genetic link, and thyroid problems tend to run in families. A predisposition may be triggered into unmistakable overactivity by several types of stress: emotional, as in a traumatic family break-up; an infection or some physical trouble; and occasionally an excess of iodine. This last may come about via the milk the child drinks, and is most likely in the first half of the year when cows are eating new spring grass, which contains more iodine than their winter fodder. The stress can set off the autoimmune type of overactive thyroid, Graves' disease, in a child who is constitutionally susceptible.

The snag is that an overactive thyroid doesn't come on in the way you might expect:

Philip was nearly expelled. His father was furious, and his mother wondered where they'd gone wrong. It all dated back to a nasty bout of streptococcal sore throat. Phil was eleven at the time, and from then on he became more and more difficult to cope with. He was always on the move and always up to something, then dreadfully upset when he was reprimanded. He had been in the top third of his class at school, but now he was near the bottom. Even his writing was sloppy and all over the place.

The woman at the child guidance clinic tried talking. Then Phil's mother had the idea that he might have worms. He was eating enormously, but was as skinny as a rake. The GP ran a battery of tests, and an excess of thyroid hormones showed up.

What you might notice in a child with overactive thyroid

Physical problems   In the younger group in particular:

- prolonged bed-wetting;
- frequent motions.

At all ages:

- neck swelling, in 95 per cent (may be slight);
- poor sleep and daytime restlessness;
- weight loss in 80 per cent;
- weight gain in 20 per cent;
- enormous appetite;
- tremor;
- itching skin, with fidgetiness;
- being tall for the child's age, but not excessively;
- being easily tired;
- weak muscles;
- mildly sore eyes, puffy lids;
- dislike of hot weather, hot rooms.

Mood and behaviour problems These may be so obvious and so troublesome that parents may hardly notice anything else going wrong, at first:

- difficulties in relationships with family members, friends and teachers;
- disruption at school – short attention span, very distractible, can't keep still;
- easily upset, bursting into tears, banging doors etc. in anger, often rude and rebellious, moody and uncooperative.

Favourable signs for recovery include an emotional stress at the beginning, a small goitre, and prompt recognition of the illness.

What is needed

When thyroid tests have confirmed that an overactive thyroid is at fault, a long course of treatment is in prospect. There are no quick miracles: the medication has to be built up gradually, and the results are gradual too. A child in this situation needs endless patience and understanding, however tiresome she may be. She is genuinely in a turmoil, and doesn't know why.

Antithyroid medicine The first step is to get the youngster established on one of the antithyroid drugs. Methimazole is preferred, since it need only be taken once a day. A more complex routine is difficult for any child to remember, let alone one with a butterfly mind from excess thyroid. The dosage is monitored by how the child feels and behaves, and after some months can often be reduced without ill effect.

About one youngster in three develops side-effects to the medication. These are not usually dangerous, but are unpleasant – for instance, feeling sick, pain in the joints, or a rash. Very occasionally a more serious problem threatens, with a sore throat or mouth ulcers (see Chapter 11). In the ordinary way the medicine is continued for one to two years before trying the effect of stopping it. If the symptoms return, the medicine must be resumed for a further year. All the time the child is on an antithyroid she, or he, must see the doctor and have a blood test every month. This can be inconvenient at times.

It is a good sign if any neck swelling is reduced during treatment, but if the goitre enlarges this indicates that the medication has been too effective and has pushed the thyroid into underactivity. This calls for a reduction in the antithyroid and/or the addition of replacement thyroxine for fine-tuning.

Radioiodine If side-effects make it uncomfortable or unsafe to continue with one antithyroid, another may be tried, but this is likely to be no better. In this case, or if a double course of antithyroid has failed to produce a lasting cure, another form of treatment must be substituted. Until five or ten years ago it was considered that radioiodine was unsuitable for growing children, in case it interfered with their development and in particular their fertility later. These fears have been proved groundless, and radioiodine is becoming the most favoured treatment for children with overactive thyroid.

Since there is no more than a 50 per cent chance of achieving satisfactory control of the disorder with antithyroid medicines, some parents and doctors together decide to go for radioiodine before any other treatment. Radioiodine is successful in 92 per cent of children, usually requiring only one dose. In nearly all cases the thyroid is switched off completely, necessitating thyroxine replacement indefinitely. This does not need frequent checking, and the frequent visits to the doctor with antithyroid treatment are avoided.

Surgery Sometimes parents feel so apprehensive about the possible adverse effects of using radioactive iodine for their child that they prefer surgery, if the antithyroid treatment is unsatisfactory. For a few days before the operation the thyroid is settled with iodine drops and the beta-blocker propranolol. Although surgery traditionally has the advantage of producing an immediate cure, it is not always completely successful – especially in children. In about a sixth of them the symptoms of overactive thyroid return some time after the operation. Then the usual choice is radioiodine after all.

Whichever specific form of treatment is used, other more general supportive measures are needed:

- super-generous nutrition, rich in protein and carbohydrate;
- extra calcium (cheese, milk, sardines);
- vitamin supplements – there may be shortages of vitamin A and the B group in particular (milk, cheese, egg yolk and carrots for A; whole wheat, pulses, eggs, liver, meat and greens for the B group).

The excess of thyroid hormones will have induced an abnormally high metabolic rate which is burning up food incredibly fast. The demand will continue for weeks after the illness itself is under control.

With so much internal as well as external activity, the child needs rest in both body and mind. A sedative may help with this. Don't be disappointed if it takes a long time for his or her mood and behaviour to calm down. This disorder is a major test for the parents, so try to make everything else as easy for yourselves as possible. You deserve it.

Eye problems

These are fairly common but never severe in children with overactive thyroid. They are likely to consist of no more than slightly sore eyes, and soothing hypromellose eyedrops are the only treatment necessary. This is not an infection like conjunctivitis.

Thyroid cancer

Cancer of the thyroid is uncommon at any age, and extremely so in childhood. Boys and girls are equally unlikely to be affected, but the risk is enhanced if the child has ever been exposed to X-rays in the neck area. Until recently X-rays were sometimes used as a treatment for acne, but this treatment has been stopped. Fortunately, thyroid cancer is a particularly mild type in children, slow-growing and with a 95 per cent cure rate. The basic symptom is a painless, hard lump in the neck which gradually gets bigger.

Treatment

Radioiodine is used in a dose sufficient to kill off the cancer cells, including any secondary spread. It incidentally prevents the healthy thyroid tissue from making its hormones, but this is easily remedied with thyroxine tablets.

Adolescents

Adolescent goitre

Adolescence is a period of great change and growth. There is a dramatic spurt in height and development, usually starting at about eleven in girls and two or three years later for boys. The reproductive organs mature, and the secondary sexual characteristics appear. They include breast development and periods in the female, and the masculine need to shave and a deepening voice. The shape and bony structure of the face and body alter too.

All this places huge demands on the metabolism, which must supply the materials for growth and the energy for building with them. Since the rate of metabolism depends on the thyroid, the gland is called upon for extra activity. It is at this stage that a goitre commonly develops. The thyroid may swell up simply because it is so busy, or it may be struggling to make the most of a supply of iodine that was borderline before, and is now inadequate for so much growth and tissue activity. One possible result, in a susceptible youngster, may be that the stress on the gland stimulates the formation of the unwanted antibodies of Hashimoto's disease. 65 per cent of adolescent goitre is due to this disorder. In most cases, at least one of the parents carries this antibody too, even if they haven't been aware of any thyroid problems.

An adolescent goitre is likely to get a little smaller over two or three years, and to remain so unless some new stress falls on the metabolism. Having a baby, an infection or physical illness, or an emotional disaster may upset the thyroid again, or a major fault in the diet may have the same effect.

Oestrogen, the female sex hormone, increases the sensitivity of the thyroid to stimulus. This accounts for the great preponderance of girls with noticeable adolescent goitres. In the seventeenth century the painter Sir Peter Lely made portraits of many of the beautiful and high-born ladies of the English court. Nearly all show the gentle outward curve of a small goitre in their necks.

Underactive and overactive thyroid problems

At this age, these problems will be due to one or other type of autoimmune disorder: Hashimoto's or Graves' types, respectively. The symptoms and signs may be any of those associated with either adult or childhood disease. The moodiness and unpredictability of teenagers may be partly due to the normal increase in T_3, the more powerful of the thyroid hormones, at this stage. If the moods become extreme, you should think about a thyroid upset. Depression and lethargy signal too little hormone, while alternating bouts of energy and exhaustion may result from too much. Either way, these youngsters are more than usually uncooperative and touchy.

The thyroid is closely involved in sexual development. Even a simple adolescent goitre often swells up seven to ten days before each period. At this key age any thyroid disturbance affects the sexual characteristics.

Lack of thyroid This usually delays the onset of puberty, but may have the opposite effect and the child becomes sexually mature, with all the physical characteristics, at eight or ten years old. Fortunately this precocious development regresses back to the normal stage with thyroid treatment. In those who have already reached puberty in the ordinary way when the thyroid deficiency shows itself, the periods become heavy, irregular and painful. Anaemia is common in hypothyroidism, due to lack of T_4, but in some girls there may also be a lack of iron from excessive losses each month.

Excess of thyroid Again, sexual development is likely to be delayed. The periods may not start up, or if they do they are liable to become scanty and to peter out. Boys remain immature with small organs for longer than their peers, and are not interested in sex.

Alison was sixteen-and-a-half when she began losing weight – far more successfully, it seemed, than the other girls at school who were into slimming. She was pleased. Her periods stopped, and she seemed to lose all her feeling for her friends. However cold it was, she would wear only the thinnest, skimpiest garments. The doctor considered several possibilities applicable to Alison's age group.

The weight loss, the lightening and loss of her periods, her awkwardness with her friends and her not feeling the cold could all add up to an overactive thyroid. On the other hand, her pleasure at losing weight and the complete absence of periods would fit in with a diagnosis of anorexia nervosa. A thyroid test showed a high level of thyroid hormones in her blood: it would have been abnormally low in anorexia.

Anorexia nervosa

This so-called slimmers' disease is most likely to affect girls between fourteen and eighteen. The key symptoms are:

- serious weight loss;
- cessation of periods;
- refusal to eat enough to keep a normal weight (in some cases deliberate vomiting to get rid of food).

The thyroid reacts to the starvation by reducing its ouput of T_4 and converting it into inactive reverse-T_3 (rT_3). This slows the metabolism, the rate at which food is used up. The heart rate slows and, because of the poor circulation, the girl's hands and feet are cold and blue. Her skin is parched, her hair is dry, and she feels deadly cold – but pleased to be losing weight. She withdraws from her friends and has near-tantrums if anyone tries to make her eat. The cause, and the cure, are psychological. She also needs a carbohydrate-based, nourishing diet. The thyroid responds rapidly to carbohydrate.

Drastic slimming, plus amphetamine or other pills

This dangerous habit affects older adolescent girls. One danger is that if there is an autoimmune tendency in the family the girl may be precipitated into Graves' disease, with a high level of thyroid hormones. Some slimming-pills contain thyroxine, and this has a direct thyrotoxic effect. The treatment involves stopping any diet pills, taking plenty of nourishment – especially protein and carbohydrate – and damping down such symptoms as tremor or palpitations with a beta-blocker for the time being. Further thyroid testing is required to assess the situation in a few weeks.

Substance abuse

Almost any of the 'social' drugs that adolescents may experiment with can cause weight loss, tremor and nerviness. The periods can be upset. This can arouse suspicions of an overactive thyroid, but tests show a normal or reduced level of the hormones. Ecstasy, crack, speed, acid and heroin can all have these effects.

Emotional stress

In this sensitive, insecure age group, whatever front they put on, emotional upsets affect adolescents greatly. Weight loss, frequent motions and passing of water, rapid pulse, sweating, tremor, poor sleep, restlessness, disrupted periods, tearfulness – all may have a psychological basis. The symptoms would fit in with overactive thyroid, but tests may exonerate the gland. Psychiatric help is then needed, often involving the parents.

Anorexia nervosa and drastic slimming with chemicals are mostly girls' problems. Drugs and emotional stress can affect either sex. For adolescents especially, psychiatric or psychological counselling and support are important when something goes wrong, whether it is a thyroid disorder or some other problem. Other treatments can run concurrently. Alison took carbimazole for a year, but still sees her therapist from time to time. She is well and happy at college.

8

The over-fifties

Thyroid problems are relatively common from fifty onwards. They matter enormously because of the mental misery and dangers to physical health they can cause. Yet they frequently go unrecognized and untreated.

The trouble is that in this age group thyroid disorders don't come over in anything like the well-defined fashion they do in younger adults. The symptoms that do appear can all be explained away easily as something quite different – for instance as part of the menopause, diabetes, high blood pressure or depression. Worst of all they may be endured without complaint as being caused simply by age: 'the sort of thing I should expect'. Then the doctor doesn't even know there is anything wrong, and cannot set off the investigations which might uncover a totally curable thyroid problem.

Just as babies, willy-nilly, are screened for thyroid abnormalities, so those of us who are middle-aged and older should have a routine thyroid check, without waiting for evidence of disease to force the issue.

In the normal way the basic metabolic rate slows down gradually over the years – you are on maintenance, not building. The amount of T_4 in the bloodstream remains much the same, but, since less is used up, less need be produced. The turnover – the time it takes to replace the stock of thyroxine – increases from seven to nine days. There is also less need, proportionately, for the super-active hormone T_3, so slightly less T_4 is converted to T_3. There is measurably less T_3 in circulation after age eighty-five.

This mild metabolic scaling-down is partly because we don't usually do as much energetic physical work or sport as we did earlier, so there is less call to burn fuel fast. Even when we are resting, the metabolic rate is more leisurely – as an economy measure and also to reduce strain on the heart and the breathing apparatus.

This doesn't mean we should accept feeling dull and lethargic or less mobile than before, but the slower metabolism does reduce the speed with which we can gear up to meet a sudden demand on muscular energy. It also makes us more vulnerable to cold. This can be an annoyance to the naturally frugal, whose instinct is to be economical with the heating.

Dick was like that: an avid turner-off of switches. Usually Judy managed, unobtrusively, to switch them on again, but things reached a crisis point when Dick retired and Judy developed an underactive thyroid. Neither of them realized what was happening, although for some time Judy had noticed that her fingers went the dead-white of Raynaud's disease whenever there was a chill in the air. Gradually she felt less and less like making any effort to keep the house warm, or indeed to do anything at all. Dick took on a lot of the energetic chores and did not notice the temperature.

During one of those cold snaps, on his return from the weekly trip to the supermarket, he found the house icy and Judy slumped in a chair, hardly aware. She was slipping into a myxoedematous coma and hypothermia. She recovered in hospital, where her thyroid deficiency was discovered. Dick? He's just the same, but now Judy is established on her T_4 supplement she is alert to the situation and keeps the house warm.

Medicines which may affect the thyroid tests

One of the features of getting into your second half-century is an increased likelihood of being on some kind of regular medication. Some medicines actually affect thyroid function directly, while others merely distort the test results.

High T_4 reading   This may be caused by:

- too high a dose of thyroxine;
- iodides in medication – for instance, cough mixtures, amiodarone (for the heart – men are especially affected), disinfectant for wounds and sores;
- oestrogens – for hormone replacement therapy, or prostate problems, or in the contraceptive pill;
- levodopa or bromocriptine – for Parkinson's disease;
- kelp – a seaweed-based health food;
- thiazide diuretics – these produce only an apparent increase in T_4, due to the loss of fluid making the blood more concentrated.

Low T_4 reading   This may be caused by:

- iodides in medication (including amiodarone and kelp – see above) switching off T_4 production instead of stimulating it;

- anti-epileptic drugs such as carbamazepine;
- diazepam (Valium);
- chlorpromazine (major tranquillizer);
- androgens and body-building steroids;
- some medicines for arthritis and rheumatism;
- salicylates, including aspirin;
- co-trimoxazole – an antibacterial drug;
- chlorpropamide and other antidiabetic drugs;
- heparin (to prevent clotting).

Reduced conversion of T_4 to T_3 T_3 readings may be reduced and T_4 may go up slightly due to the effects of beta-blockers such as propranolol, nadolol and stanozolol.

In the over-fifties, test results are much more subject to day-to-day variation, whether or not any medicine is being taken. Repeat tests may be necessary to check inconsistent readings (see also Chapter 10).

Underactive thyroid

This condition is increasingly prevalent from age fifty, and is fourteen times as likely in a woman as a man. The chances of developing it are around 5 per cent per year if we carry the antithyroid antibodies in our blood – and nearly 1 in 5 of us do so, without ever having had any thyroid problems. Some people become hypothyroid as the end result of treatment with radioiodine or surgery for Graves' disease, maybe years earlier. For others it may be the effect of one of the medicines mentioned above. For the majority it will be a late, slow development of Hashimoto's disease – a reaction to abnormal antibodies.

It is important not to ignore any pointers to thyroid lack for fear of being a nuisance or making a fuss about nothing. Of course there may be other reasons for what you notice, but if it is a thyroid problem it needs treatment.

What to look out for

Physical symptoms These may include the following:

- *Slowing down* Everything takes twice as long.
- *Constipation* This is never due to age alone, but can be brought on by too little exercise, not drinking enough, and medicines such as cold cures and antidepressants – or too little thyroid.

- *Loss of weight* This is in contrast to the gain which is typical of underactive thyroid at other ages. Your appetite is down, too.
- *Your face looks older* over a matter of months, and is also sallow and puffy, without its normal expressiveness. Your nearest and dearest are likely to notice it, and to worry.
- *Your hair gets thinner* and finer, but instead of going grey tends towards a dull, darkish hue. An odd point: you lose the outer third of each eyebrow.
- *Raynaud's disease* Like Judy (page 91), your fingers may go dead and pale even with slight cold. They recover painfully when you warm them up.
- *Deafness* You may become increasingly hard of hearing, and also suffer from vertigo and the constant whistling in the ears called tinnitus. It is all due to thyroid deprivation affecting the hearing and balance nerves.
- *Your voice* becomes hoarse, and it isn't the normal effect of maturity. Friends will be more aware of this than you.
- *Cholesterol-clogging* of your blood vessels, leading to angina (chest pain with exercise), faints, fits, and shortness of breath. In the ordinary way the thyroid hormones work to keep the cholesterol in circulation at a lower level.
- *Anaemia* This can be due to lack of thyroxine, and compounds the problem of clogged arteries by reducing the quality of the blood that does get through.
- *Heart problems* These are the most likely reason for you to consult your doctor if you have an underactive thyroid starting from fifty-plus. The rhythm of the heartbeat may be disturbed, which makes the heart pump inefficiently. This in turn leads to congestion in the body, with swelling ankles and shortness of breath. Anginal chest pain can increase, coming even when you are resting, and your blood pressure may go up, but not seriously.

    A snag is that the start of treatment may make matters worse. Your heart may have been able to cope with the slowed-down metabolism and heart rate of too little thyroid, but is put under strain when there is an all-round speed-up. The answer is a two-pronged treatment: thyroxine, which is necessary to rescue your general health from deterioration, and propranolol or digoxin to protect your heart from overworking too hard.
- *Rheumatic problems* Commonest are muscular weakness and 'rheumaticky' aching, especially in the neck. Although your muscles don't look smaller, and may even be slightly bigger, there is a loss of active, working muscle cells, made up for in bulk

with packing material. Arthritis, causing muscle pain, may affect little joints, but lack of thyroxine seldom involves knees and hips. Gout, rheumatoid arthritis and polymyalgia are all more likely in sufferers from Hashimoto's autoimmune type of thyroid under-activity. So is the carpal-tunnel syndrome, which is recognized by pins and needles in the hands (see page 31).

- *Goitre* This is not likely to be a feature in the fifty-plus age group, and any long-standing swelling will probably have shrunk, if anything.

Mental and emotional symptoms The symptoms which show them-selves in your mood, personality, and mental speed and efficiency are often the most distressing to endure. Added to this, other people tend to regard them with impatience, rather than offering the help and sympathy that physical disorders attract. Psychological changes may also be not only the worst but the first to appear.

From your point of view, you find yourself inexplicably less alert and confident. You have lost all interest, let alone enthusiasm, in your favourite activities. You can't seem to care about the people who mean most to you. You may feel pointlessly agitated, hopelessly indecisive, or just empty. Your memory and concentra-tion are apt to be erratic, and you can't deal with the sort of problems you would have sailed through before. You sleep for a long time and may drop off in the day, but you never feel refreshed. This is because you are missing out on 'Stage-4' sleep – the deepest and most reviving part.

All this could add up to a severe depressive illness, while relatives may be thinking of Alzheimer's disease. If the problem is an underactive thyroid, antidepressants will be useless and will make any constipation worse, but the thyroid tests will be positive. This is the signal to start thyroxine treatment gently.

Since the shortage of thyroid will have built up over many months, during the recovery period you will seem to grow younger, miraculously. You will be livelier, happier, more mobile week by week. Your feelings of affection will come out of the deep-freeze, as will your ability to think and work things out. You will have to remain on the tablets indefinitely, but this is a small price to be your proper self. At your age the dosage need not be large, but without it you would be at risk of degenerating into an immobile, brainless lump.

Since the treatment of underactive thyroid is so simple and magically effective, it would be a tragedy not to have it. If you are developing the disorder you may have several or only one of the pointers to the possibility. If there's any question, the sensible move is to go along for a check. You've nothing to lose, much to gain.

Myxoedema

Myxoedema is the ultimate stage in underactive thyroid, named after the typical puffiness (oedema) of the skin, as well as the other signs and symptoms of thyroid deficiency. There are likely to be problems in the nervous system particularly, including pins and needles anywhere in the body. Unsteadiness, with a real risk of falls, results from thyroid lack in the cerebellum – the part of the brain that coordinates movement. Myxoedema is unlikely in the younger age groups.

Myxoedema coma   This dangerous slide into unconsciousness most often affects women who are definitely elderly – seventy-five-plus – and living alone. The final precipitant that brings it on is often another illness, such as a bladder or chest infection. Alcohol, sedatives or such major tranquillizers as chlorpromazine increase the risk, as does neglect of nourishment, warmth and comfort. The body temperature may fall too low for an ordinary clinical thermometer to register.

This is the way Dick's wife, Judy, was heading. She was lucky he came in when he did, since even today this development carries a high mortality. Back in 1961 only 1 in 5 recovered.

The treatment consists in gradual rewarming, with blankets in a room of normal temperature, urgent T_4 or T_3 by injection or in a tube to the stomach, antibiotics and sometimes steroids temporarily.

Myxoedema madness   With myxoedema the chances are that a friend or relative will see that something is dreadfully wrong, rather than the sufferer herself. This is particularly true of the serious psychiatric upset that can be part of the illness. While usually the victim is profoundly lethargic and depressed, she may be irrational or even delirious, but more likely feels persecuted, suspecting plots and deadly threats from neighbours, acquaintances, television or the government. Reason and reassurance are useless: psychiatric help is essential, preferably in a hospital where the whole illness can be brought under control.

Men very rarely slip into serious myxoedema, partly because they are in general less vulnerable to thyroid disorders, but also because men of any age are often cared for by someone else. Their illness would be nipped in the bud.

Overactive thyroid

The chances of having an overactive thyroid increase with age: 10 per cent of all cases crop up in the over-seventies. Around eight times as many women as men are affected – a lower proportion than for the underactive group. In fact 2 per cent of women of sixty and over are known to be suffering from too much thyroid hormone, apart from those undiagnosed. How many of your thin, agitated and inefficient middle-aged acquaintances are struggling with an overload of T_4?

Four out of five whose thyroids become overactive at this age are harbouring the peculiar thyroid-stimulating antibodies of Graves' disease. At least half of them have no detectable goitre; a few have a smooth, all-over swelling; and the rest have a long-standing, knobbly, multinodular goitre which has started playing up, perhaps in only one nodule.

The occasional causes include the early phase of de Quervain's inflammation of the thyroid (page 24), hashitoxicosis (page 53), or the effect of medication (see the list on pages 109–11). Men are especially vulnerable to a reaction with amiodarone. Trouble from this useful drug cannot be dealt with just by stopping it, since it lurks in the system for months. Beta-blockers are the first line of defence while a strategy for both heart and thyroid is worked out.

What to look out for

Just as with too little thyroid, too much produces very different effects after fifty compared with earlier.

Heart disorder   This is the major group of symptoms, often the first to appear, and vitally important. It shows up in:

- palpitations;
- rapid, irregular pulse – atrial fibrillation;
- tight, choking chest pain with exertion – angina;
- breathlessness with the slightest effort;
- swollen ankles;
- mauvish complexion at times;
- exhaustion;
- faints;
- raised blood pressure.

The give-away feature is a disappointing lack of improvement in the symptoms with the usual heart drugs, unless the excess thyroid is also corrected.

Apathetic thyrotoxicosis Among those of us over fifty, a sizeable minority reacts to too much thyroid with the opposite of the usual symptoms:

Regular type	*Apathetic type*
Peak age forty-plus	Peak age sixty-seven
Big appetite	No appetite, nausea
Frequent motions	Constipation
Anxiety	Depression, apathy
Restlessness	Lethargy
Comes on over months	Takes several years

Other Symptoms In both regular and apathetic thyrotoxicosis, look out for:

- severe weight loss – of from 10 lb to 2 stone;
- worsening of asthma or other breathing problems;
- warm skin, but not sweaty at this age;
- fatigue;
- uneasy, unrefreshing sleep;
- extreme weakness of the big muscles, with pain and stiffness;
- 'frozen shoulder' from inflammation of the covering of the joint;
- thinning of the bones, with a risk of fracture.

Occasionally there may also be:

- prominent eyes – these are less likely at this age, but can be caused by airways disease, not the thyroid;
- thickening and purplish-red discolouration of the skin over the shins.

What to do

The first essential is to pinpoint what precisely is at fault, by the standard blood tests for thyroid hormones, possibly a scintigram, and, in the case of a single nodule, a fine-needle aspiration (see Chapter 11). If you have heart symptoms you may need a beta-blocker or digoxin or both, as well as the treatment for overactive thyroid. Radioiodine is the preferred treatment, with surgery second, since in middle age there is more risk of side-effects with protracted use of the antithyroid drugs such as carbimazole.

The thyroid, in common with other parts of your body, needs to be treated with consideration at this age. That means a short course of a beta-blocker with an antithyroid if necessary to calm the overactivity down before either of the two major treatments.

If you have a long-standing goitre it is essential to have one of the permanent, curative processes, but if you have Graves' auto-immune disorder with no noticeable goitre or only a small, smooth swelling, there's the slight chance that the disorder will die down with a short course of antithyroid and not relapse.

Laura and Elspeth are sisters, not very much alike and with five years between them. At the time it all started, each was worried about the other. Laura, the elder, looked dreadful. She had lost so much weight that her clothes hung on her as though she were a coat-hanger, and, in spite of pressure from her husband and her sister, she picked at her food and ate next to nothing. Laura herself was worried, but she wouldn't go to the doctor because she was afraid of what she might be told. Anyway, she felt too tired to bother. She'd read somewhere that sixty to seventy was the cancer decade, and everyone knows that you lose weight with cancer.

It was only when the doctor came to check on Laura's eighty-five-year-old mother that he noticed how thin Laura was, and her agitated manner. He insisted, in the kindest way, on running the rule over her at the surgery. Her overactive thyroid came to light, and she was soon on the road to recovery.

Elspeth also had a thyroid problem. She'd had a goitre for years, but it didn't give her any trouble so she ignored it. She'd always been overweight, and tried to eat sensibly, but she now seemed to feel hungry all the time. This wasn't why she went to see the doctor – the problems bothering her were feeling so tired, getting short of breath, and her ankles ballooning up. The doctor listened to her heart and did an electrocardiogram. Together with her fast, irregular heartbeat, the electrical recording showed that she had atrial fibrillation. This, together with her being overweight, would certainly account for her symptoms, but the goitre and her being told that there were thyroid problems in the family reminded the doctor to ask some more questions, and to send her off for a blood test.

She – Elspeth's GP – was interested to hear that Laura had waves of anxiety, which were not like her proper self, especially with no reason. The test result showed that, although the effects had been quite different, Elspeth had an excess of thyroid hormone, like Laura's a few months before. Because of Elspeth's heart condition, the doctor was particularly careful to reduce the heart strain and excess of T_4 gradually, before giving her radioiodine. If the goitre had been awkwardly big, or there had been a single, particularly large nodule, the choice would have veered towards surgery.

Both sisters now have to take thyroxine daily, since a few months after radioiodine treatment, but this is a small inconvenience to keep in good health.

Cancer

From fifty upwards, anyone who finds a lump in their neck or anywhere else thinks of cancer. Even if there isn't anything new but an increase in size of part of a goitre you've had for years, it is a worry that needs sorting out. The least worrying kind is the general lumpiness of an established multinodular goitre.

If there is a tumour, a scintigram will show it up and will give an indication of its type – there are several thyroid varieties. Fine-needle aspiration is especially useful for checking out a single suspicious nodule. (See Chapter 11 for details of both these techniques.) For the best results, it is important to find out the situation and start whatever treatment is appropriate without delay.

Between ages sixty and sixty-nine the risk of a thyroid cancer is 3½ in 100,000; it becomes less after eighty. Most thyroid cancers are very slow-growing, and often a thyroid cancer is discovered only after the person has died of something else. Apart from an enlarging lump, the only symptoms, if any, may be hoarseness without a sore throat, and very rarely some discomfort in swallowing.

Treatment

Some types of thyroid cancer are best treated by an operation, followed by radioiodine, but radioiodine alone is usually all that is necessary. A sizeable dose is used, which knocks out the good as well as the bad thyroid cells, so you have to take thyroxine for ever afterwards. The results are excellent.

Other illnesses

It is more likely now than earlier in your life that you will have acquired some signs of wear and tear of bodily flaws. They may have no relation to your thyroid, but they need care in their own right. They may also cause symptoms which you might think are due to thyroid. For instance, it is commonplace to develop diabetes in middle age, and this can cause lassitude. Coronary or rheumatic heart disease can develop with a perfect thyroid, as can arthritis of any type, bronchitis and emphysema.

While your thyroid can be upset temporarily by an acute illness like flu or shingles, it will right itself automatically. Even long-lasting problems are only likely to put your thyroid out of kilter through the medicines you may have to take – see pages 109–11. The good thing about a thyroid problem is that it can nearly always be put right and leaves no lasting damage.

9

The other thyroid hormone

Most of us think of the thyroid hormones as T_4 and T_3, which control our metabolism. But they are not the whole story. About thirty years ago another thyroid hormone, 'calcitonin', was discovered. It is made in the thyroid gland by some special cells – the 'C' cells.

Calcitonin affects the way the body deals with calcium, the important mineral in bones and teeth. Calcium is also vital for the working of the automatic muscles – for instance your bowels, your bladder and, essentially, your heart. Too much or too little calcium in the blood can literally be fatal. The bones are used as a handy, on-the-spot repository for excess calcium, and the kidneys wash out any surplus via the urine.

The calcium level is largely controlled by the parathyroid glands, four little chunks of tissue attached to the back of the thyroid lobes. They produce their own special hormone to do this, but they are relatively slow to react to changes in the amount of calcium in circulation, taking three or four hours. This is where calcitonin from the thyroid steps in. The 'C' cells respond within minutes if the calcium level goes up 10 per cent. They can rev up calcitonin production to six times the normal.

This process comes into action in the ordinary way after a meal, especially one including plenty of calcium (from cheese, milk, yoghurt or sardines, for example). Under the influence of the surge of calcitonin, appetite is switched off almost immediately and the blood is cleared of excess calcium by dumping the surplus into the bones. Within an hour, and continuing for several days, extra bone-building cells are produced, to organize the extra calcium, but in the longer term calcitonin slows down bone turnover.

Paget's disease

Bones, like other tissues, are constantly being replaced and renewed. In Paget's disease, which affects elderly men more than women, bone turnover is too fast. Because of all this activity, the affected bones feel warm through the skin and they grow bigger and clumsily shaped. Those likeliest to be involved include the shin and thigh bones, the pelvis and the skull (where pressure by the enlarged bone on the hearing nerve can cause deafness).

Reggie had a headache – a deep ache right in the bones of his forehead – and his cap seemed too tight. He had a bit of a pain in his left shin as well. He was sixty-six. The doctor told him he had Paget's disease, and there was nothing to worry about. Reggie was not satisfied: 'But it hurts, and the ordinary painkillers like aspirin and Nurofen don't touch it.' The most effective way of stopping the pain of Paget's is an injection of calcitonin.

Too much calcium in the blood (hypercalcaemia)

Calcitonin injections are also useful in this condition. It may develop in Graves' disease because of the disturbed metabolism, in anyone bedbound for months, with the prolonged use of certain water tablets (thiazide diuretics), or as a result of excess of vitamin D prescribed for medical reasons. Very occasionally someone with an underactive thyroid may have such a sluggish metabolism that calcium isn't moved on through its normal cycle but builds up in the blood.

In young people too much calcium can lead to kidney stones, with acute pain, but in older age groups the symptoms are very different, and vague. There is fatigue for no reason, weakness, low spirits and a sense of not feeling 'up to the mark'. Often the sufferer doesn't realize how poorly he has been until treatment with calcitonin restores him to his normal self.

Osteoporosis

This weakening of the bones, with a propensity to fracture, is increasingly common after forty, especially in women. Typically, it develops when oestrogen levels are drastically cut by the menopause or by operations on the ovaries. At the same time, calcitonin levels are reduced. This is thought to be one of the causes of the disorder. Calcitonin treatment may be useful. Hormone replacement therapy (HRT) is effective, but some people cannot take it because of breast or womb conditions, a clotting tendency, or high blood pressure. The snag about calcitonin is that to treat osteoporosis it must be given by injection, at least three times a week, and a course lasts six months. It is also expensive. Etidronate by mouth is not as effective, but it is the best alternative available at present.

Too little calcium in the blood
(hypocalcaemia)

The parathyroid glands are intimately close neighbours of the thyroid, but quite separate. They lie behind the thyroid gland, two on each side, and each weighs about an ounce. Their delicate blood vessels run across the back of the thyroid and can easily be damaged during an operation for a goitre or tumour.

Damage to the parathyroids, directly or through the blood supply, causes symptoms within days. The level of calcium in the blood falls too low, and this leads to pins and needles round the mouth, tinglings, and intense anxiety. Muscle cramps, spasms and ultimately convulsions follow – rather like the effects of hyperventilation. If the symptoms persist, a few weeks on calcium tablets will resolve the situation before they become severe.

The parathyroids are likely to have been only slightly bruised or irritated by the thyroid operation. In the rare circumstance of permanent parathyroid lack, calcitriol capsules, containing a synthetic vitamin-D preparation, are required. Checks of the calcium level must be made regularly.

Apart from parathyroid damage, hypocalcaemia – too little calcium in the blood – can result from:

- long-term use of oestrogen-containing HRT or the Pill;
- diuretics such as frusemide, which may wash too much calcium out in the water;
- some kidney problems;
- anticonvulsant medicines, and some tranquillizers;
- diet – not enough calcium (dairy foods), or excess of wholewheat and other cereals which hinder the absorption of calcium.

10

Keeping your thyroid happy

Your thyroid is an obliging organ. You can anticipate a lifetime of trouble-free service at minimal cost to you. It will organize the intricate working of your whole body to fit changing circumstances. It will make swift adjustments in the face of illness, injury or disaster, much as a car with an automatic gearbox will respond to driving conditions, without your having to do anything. The thyroid, however, runs a more complicated machine and is far more sensitive. It will make immediate, medium- and long-term alterations to your metabolism according to what you eat, how much you use your muscles, your mood, your age and any stresses you are under – and even the weather.

What does this remarkable and priceless piece of equipment require to keep running? Its demands could not be more modest: an average Western diet and a supply of clean drinking water. The ingredients of your food which are of special concern to the thyroid are iodine, a vital element, which no other hormones use, and various vitamins.

Iodine

A minute amount of iodine is sufficient, while an excess is harmful. The thyroid gland can store up iodine to last for two or three months, but the daily requirement averages out at about 90 micrograms (90 mcg). Less than 50 mcg throws a strain on the thyroid. One response it makes is to switch production in favour of T_3 instead of the usual 90 per cent T_4, since one molecule of T_3 needs only three-quarters as much iodine as one of T_4. In the UK the usual diet provides 100 to 150 mcg, but in the USA it ranges from 100 to 600 mcg. Micrograms are minute: a small carton of yoghurt contains about 125 grams – that is, 125,000,000 micrograms.

Sources of iodine for most of us

- Dairy products – 56 per cent (this is at a maximum in the spring and summer months).
- Bread and cereals – 16 per cent.

- Meat and fish, especially sea fish and shellfish – 11 per cent.
- Sugar – 11 per cent.
- Drinks – 4 per cent.

If you live by the sea, you will even get some iodine from the air you breathe, but the water supply and locally grown vegetables will provide a negligible amount. There is a coastal area in Wales where the population used to be chronically short of iodine, due to the poor quality of the soil, like that in mountainous districts. In some countries and some states in America, very small amounts of iodine are added to the salt or the flour. This is not thought to be necessary in Britain, although some people prefer to use sea salt in the home.

Unless you live in a remote area, where goitre is obviously prevalent, and all your food is produced on the spot, you won't actually have to worry about getting enough iodine. In some circumstances, however, you need to make extra sure of your supply – for instance at the female crunch points of puberty, pregnancy and the change. This also applies to anyone after a physical illness, especially in the winter, or a period of overactive thyroid. A prolonged cold spell makes the thyroid work harder, which means it uses more of its raw materials. The safe ploy is to have two sea fish meals a week. The top natural provider of iodine is halibut – fresh or smoked – with whiting a poor second, and herring in third place. If you really can't stand fish, go for the dairy products – yoghurt, cheese, butter and milk.

Vitamins

The other dietary requirement for the thyroid more than other organs is an adequate supply of most vitamins. Again, this is especially important for the same key groups that need a little more iodine than usual. As with iodine, excess of many vitamins can be as damaging as not enough. Your aim must be to obtain them safely via your food, not through synthetic concentrates.

Which vitamins and where to find them

Vitamin A   Go for yellow – carrots, cheese, butter or margarine, egg yolk, fresh apricots and, the exception, green vegetables. The thyroid has a special relationship with this vitamin. Without the thyroid hormone your body cannot deal with vitamin A properly, and you develop an all-over yellowish tinge. This sometimes occurs in severe anorexia nervosa, when the hormone level is right down.

The B-group vitamins There are several requirements in this group:

- *Thiamine* This is found in whole wheat, pulses, nuts and pork, but rice, white flour and raw fish interfere with your being able to use it. The thyroid needs this vitamin to organize the metabolism of carbohydrates, our staple food.
- *Riboflavin* This is found in liver, cheese and eggs, or meat and yeast extracts.
- *Niacin* This is found in liver, kidneys, eggs, yeast extract and instant coffee.
- *Vitamin B12* Meat, poultry, liver, eggs and milk. Beware of running low on this one if you are a vegetarian, and especially if there is any autoimmune illness in the family. The resulting pernicious anaemia is frequently found in sufferers from Hashimoto's and Graves' diseases.
- *Vitamin B6* This is available in almost all foods. The biggest danger is accidentally overdosing with vitamin pills.

Vitamin C Citrus fruits, peppers, salads, green vegetables. You need this one in particular to pep up your immune system – which is all the more vital if you have been exposed to any form of stress.

Vitamin D Herrings (including kippers), sardines, margarine and eggs plus a regular dose of sunshine. If you are dark, you need more sun than a blonde to manufacture the vitamin in your skin. Unless you are specifically advised by your doctor, don't go for fish-liver oils or pills – too much vitamin D is definitely dangerous.

Vitamin E Margarine, sunflower seed oil and other polyunsaturates, wheatgerm. No one runs short of this one unless they are actually starving.

The only other basic to keep your thyroid happy is clean, uncontaminated drinking water – something most of us can take for granted. Localized outbreaks of goitre and thyroid failure have occurred in various parts of Europe from time to time. They have been traced to pollution with sewage, confined to those sharing the same water supply. Michelangelo may have been right to blame his goitre on the 'stagnant streams' of the Sistine Chapel.

Diets that upset the thyroid

Chronic overeating

A brief binge, especially of the sweet-tooth variety, sets the thyroid off into releasing extra T_3. This speeds up the metabolism for an hour or so, and does something towards using up the excess.

In response to continued overeating, however, the thyroid goes on producing more T_3. The increased rate of metabolism throws a strain on the heart, circulation and breathing apparatus. You know that you are overstepping the mark if your heart starts hammering and you are uncomfortably hot and slightly short of breath.

The rev-up happens only while you are still overloading your body with nourishment: it is not affected by your actual weight. You can be 20 stone, but now eating an average diet, with a stationary weight, and your thyroid won't react at all: your metabolic rate will be normal.

Undernutrition

While overeating puts a mild strain on your thyroid, eating too little really upsets it. If you start on a slimming jag or for some other reason you suddenly cut down drastically, within a day or two your thyroid has responded. It starts converting T_4 into inactive reverse-T_3 instead of the active hormone. The effect is an immediate reduction in the rate at which the body burns up its nourishment.

You are likely to feel cold, and, because of the effect on your heart rate and circulation, you may develop a headache. You may have noticed this at the beginning of dieting or if you miss several meals consecutively for other reasons. As little as 1½ oz of biscuit, bread or a banana will put you right straightaway. If you continue on a restricted diet, your body resets to a lower basic metabolic rate, to allow it to run economically on whatever nourishment is available.

It is T_3 that actually controls the metabolism, from T_4 which has been converted. Initially, while T_3 levels are down, your T_4 output stays near normal for some time. Finally, if there is still a food shortage, T_4 output is reduced too. The mental and physical slowdown of underactive thyroid then comes into effect.

The key to recovery is a carbohydrate diet. An 800 kcal meal – say pizza and apple pie – gives you a flying start towards normal thyroid function. A fatty diet may fill you up but does nothing to restore normality to your metabolism. A high-protein diet is only slightly better than this, probably because the body can make sugar out of protein, though not from fat.

It was pasta that put Stephen back on track. He had been anxious about his finals, plus his girlfriend had defected. From then on he practically lived on black coffee. He didn't fancy eating, anyway. Instead of being right on the ball, he felt dopey and couldn't concentrate on the mass of revision he knew he must do. His friend Bernie saved the day by looking in to see where Stephen had got to, and bringing with him a pasta dish he'd made, with a Danish pastry to follow.

The spell was broken. Stephen felt less lethargic, less depressed, and hungry again for the normal diet of a student on a grant – with plenty of carbohydrate filler. He did scrape through the exams.

Too much iodine

This is a rarity from ordinary food. The exceptions have been hamburgers made from the neck of the animal, probably including some thyroid gland accidentally. After several outbreaks of thyroid and iodine-excess symptoms in the American Mid-West, neck meat is not now used for ground-beef products. In Hokkaido, Japan, where the population were in the habit of eating a seaweed called kombu, overdosage of iodine led to goitres and a switch-off of thyroid hormone production.

Although there may be a brief burst of thyroid overactivity, the usual outcome of iodine excess is to suppress the thyroid. Cows fed on sea-kale can concentrate the iodine in their milk, and this has caused thyroid upsets in children. The use of iodized disinfectants in dairy work has also caused problems.

To all intents and purposes there is a negligible chance of taking in too much iodine through ordinary food in the West. Special slimmers' meals and drinks, however, often contain excessive amounts of iodine, which could cause trouble if you used them too enthusiastically. Health-food shops supply kelp, a seaweed rich in iodine, and multivitamin/multimineral preparations which can poison the thyroids of health freaks.

An iodine-reducing diet, sometimes needed before a whole-body scan in suspected cancer, involves avoiding:

- iodized or sea salt;
- milk and dairy products;
- eggs;
- seafood;
- kelp tablets etc.;
- red food dyes (erythrosine).

Foods that prevent the thyroid from using available iodine

These are called goitrogens, because eating them freely leads to goitre and the symptoms of underactive thyroid. They are all plant foods:

- cabbage and many other members of the brassica family – sprouts, cauliflower, kohlrabi, horseradish;
- peanuts, walnuts, almonds;
- rape and mustard seed;
- maize (sweet corn), millet, sorghum;
- soya – especially as part of a high-fibre diet, since too much thyroid hormone and iodine are excreted from the body;
- cassava – a major problem in Third World countries;
- also kale, raw swedes and turnips fed to cattle and coming through in their milk, as has occurred in the UK.

These plants contain cyanide derivatives which prevent the thyroid from taking in enough iodine. Matters are made worse if you use a lot of salt. The thyroid swells as it struggles to do its work.

The only people likely to run into trouble with goitrogens are the vulnerable groups, children who have less variety in the diet than we do, and health enthusiasts. Moderation is the safe watchword, and risks arise if you have a craze for nuts and soya instead of more commonplace sources of protein. The goitrogens have done us a good turn, however: the original antithyroid drugs, so useful in Graves' disease, were developed through these plants.

Medicines that can cause problems

Medicines that can strain your thyroid

Any of the following can interfere with the smooth working of the gland, or at least upset the tests:

- tolbutamide (Rastinon), for diabetes;
- chlorpropamide (Diabinese), also for diabetes;
- phenylbutazone (Butacote), for ankylosing spondylitis;
- diazepam (Valium), for anxiety;
- heparin, to prevent clotting in heart problems;
- lithium (Priadel), to prevent relapse in psychiatric illness. More than a third of people taking lithium develop an underactive thyroid;
- beta-blockers (e.g. Inderal), for high blood pressure;
- salicylates, including aspirin (e.g. Disprin), a pain-killer;

- steroids (e.g. prednisolone), for any severe physical reaction;
- phenothiazines (e.g. Largactil), major tranquillizers;
- amiloride (e.g. Moduretic), a water tablet;
- androgens (e.g. testosterone), male sex hormone;
- tamoxifen, an anti-oestrogen to ward off breast cancer;
- sulphonamides, anti-bacterial drugs;
- acetazolamide (Diamox), for glaucoma and fluid retention;
- resorcinol (Anusol), used for piles;
- PAS, for tuberculosis.

All of these medicines suppress thyroid activity, so that the level of T_4 in the blood is low, even if the gland is perfectly healthy. Sometimes, particularly with lithium, long-term thyroid lack of the Hashimoto type develops.

The following medicines have a different effect:

- phenytoin and related medicines – these anticonvulsants, used to control epilepsy, use up the thyroid hormones unusually quickly, and this may cause a shortage;
- carbamazepine (Tegretol) – this anticonvulsant inhibits the release of T_4 into the blood;
- co-trimoxazole (Septrin) – for urinary infections – also inhibits the release of T_4 into the blood;
- levodopa (Sinemet) and bromocriptine (Parlodel) are both used for Parkinson's disease, and both stop the stimulating action of TSH, leading to T_4 and T_3 lack.

Medicines that seem to increase T_4 and T_3

Although neither actually stimulates the production of more hormones:

- oestrogen (in the contraceptive pill and HRT), provides more of the transport protein;
- frusemide-type water tablets (e.g. Lasix), by getting rid of fluid, make the blood more concentrated so there is more of the hormones per millilitre.

Medicines containing iodine

Be wary of these if you have ever had a thyroid problem, and think if it could be your thyroid if you get some puzzling symptoms when you are taking one of them. These medicines are liable to give your thyroid more iodine than it can cope with. It may react by going into overdrive and producing too much hormone, with anxiety and palpitations in consequence, especially to start with. The usual end result, however, is near-complete downing of tools by the gland so that it runs into obvious underactivity, and general bodily slowing up.

- *Amiodarone (Cordarone X)* is an excellent medicine for tricky faults in the rhythm of the heart, but it causes thyroid problems in 6 per cent of people taking it. These may be due to either under- or overactivity, with totally different symptoms: snail-pace or edgy speed. Since it takes a long time to clear amiodarone from the circulation, and anyway it may be vital for the heart, it is usually best to continue with it, but help the thyroid with other drugs. These will be thyroxine in the case of underactivity, or an antithyroid such as carbimazole in the opposite situation.
- *Cough medicines* containing iodides – including over-the-counter preparations – are not for you if you've ever had a thyroid problem.
- *X-ray contrast media,* given for instance for gall-bladder investigations.
- *Povidone skin antiseptic (Betadine) and tincture of iodine* Very little iodine is likely to get into the system from these but they should be avoided during pregnancy.
- *Multivitamin/multimineral health pills.*

Your genes

Of course you cannot choose your parents or the genes they donate to you, even to make your thyroid happy. For sure you won't have the dreadful legacy of a famous family of travelling tinkers, who ranged round Scotland two hundred years ago. They intermarried and all had huge goitres and deficient thyroids. For us, it is useful to know what illnesses other family members have had. The closer the relationship, the more relevant. Any kind of thyroid disorder is important, especially since the major forms – Graves' and Hashimoto's – are due to an autoimmune process. Other auto-immune disorders indicate a tendency to react to stress by making antibodies against the body's own tissues, including the thyroid. Autoimmune conditions to look out for are:

- vitiligo – a patchy loss of pigment in the skin;
- diabetes – the type that requires insulin;
- rheumatoid arthritis;
- pernicious anaemia;
- myasthenia gravis – a rare muscle weakness;
- lupus;
- Parkinson's disease.

111

Even if one of these problems is present in your family, you are by no means bound to develop it or a thyroid disorder. It is a useful reminder to give your thyroid consideration, however, and to be alert for symptoms, especially the vague ones, that could mean that the gland is in difficulties. As we've seen, there is effective treatment for most thyroid problems. The important thing is to recognize the possibility of a thyroid disorder and have a check, especially if you are on any of the medicines or have a partiality for any of the foods known to upset the thyroid.

Of course, avoid stress, if you can.

Stress

This term can refer to a range of quite different situations. What they have in common is that something must give – mind or body. The effect may be mild and short-lived or may develop into a definite illness.

Stresses that can affect the thyroid:

- starvation, as in anorexia nervosa or drastic slimming;
- a road-traffic or similar serious accident;
- surgical operation;
- severe burns;
- radiation, for treatment or by accident;
- emotional upset, such as bereavement;
- important exams;
- major psychiatric illness, such as schizophrenia, mania or severe depression – but not Alzheimer's disease or being a psychopath, nor neurotic problems;
- great restriction of freedom, as in prison;
- withdrawal symptoms for heroin or alcohol;
- taking amphetamines or Ecstasy;
- physical illness – you can expect the thyroid to bounce back to normal as soon as your body does, except when the liver or kidneys are involved.

All these stresses can rock the thyroid, calling forth at first an extra release of thyroxine, both free and the less immediately available part attached to its carrier protein. This is the stress syndrome. It can trigger Graves' disease, but probably only if you already have the antibodies in your blood, and the disorder would have happened at some time anyway.

The boost effect of stress may be followed by a down-swing in thyroid activity. For example, during an operation the levels of T_4

and T_3 shoot up, but afterwards they slip below normal, temporarily. There are two specific stress hormones: adrenalin and cortisol. Adrenalin is the first-line response, and it stimulates the thyroid as well as pepping you up in general. Ongoing stress leads to the production of high levels of cortisol, your body's own steroid. Like steroid medicines, it suppresses thyroid activity, and in anyone already vulnerable the underactivity may persist.

In most cases your thyroid helps you through the stress and then returns to normal.

A whole group of stressful circumstances arise in the various physical illnesses. They affect the thyroid in slightly different ways.

Feverish illness   Any illness that raises your body temperature will make the thyroid produce inactive reverse-T_3 instead of the effective hormone. This slows down the rate at which you burn up your food, which is helpful when you are already too hot and don't feel like eating much.

Common illnesses such as cystitis, bronchitis, tummy upsets and flu, all lead to the low-T_3 syndrome. Less T_4 is changed into active T_3. This tends to conserve your energy, and does not mean any fault in the thyroid. If you notice undue lethargy and inability to concentrate lingering after flu or some other viral illness, there is just the faintest chance that Hashimoto's thyroiditis is starting up. However, it is much more likely to be the tag end of your body's and your thyroid's reaction to the infection. Tests would confirm this.

Serious illnesses, either acute or long-term – such as pneumonia, a coronary heart attack, cancer, especially of the lung, severe anorexia nervosa, diabetes or alcoholism – all cause a reduction in both the thyroid hormones. You may get some of the symptoms of underactive thyroid. You may look pale, feel cold and listless, and slow down mentally. These effects are likely to be noticeable in several conditions.

HIV   The infection alone causes no reaction in the thyroid, but in ARC – AIDS-related complex, comprising fatigue, enlarged glands and diarrhoea – T_4 is increased but T_3 reduced. The net effect is a slightly lower metabolic rate, to add to the lack of vitality. In full AIDS, when the illness has tightened its grip, levels of both hormones are down and no part of the body is working properly.

Heroin, methadone or other narcotic abuse, depending on its severity, has a similar effect of all-over slowly grinding to a halt.

These reactions by the thyroid reduce the demands on the heart and other parts of the body, which is generally helpful during a bad illness. There is no need, no point, in trying to correct the lack of thyroid – everything reverts to normal when the physical illness improves sufficiently.

There are a few exceptions, however:

Chronic diarrhoea, from whatever cause, depletes the body of thyroid hormones faster than the gland can replace them. This is a forced shortage of thyroid, not a reaction to illness, and it is reasonable to use thyroxine tablets while the bowel trouble is sorted out.

Liver disorders Some types of inflammation of the liver – hepatitis – cause a brief increase in T_4 in the circulation. The liver manufactures the protein that carries T_4 round in the blood, and when it is irritated it may release more of this protein than usual. It could make you feel unexpectedly restless during the illness, but it is a temporary effect. Serious liver problems, such as alcoholic cirrhosis, put the thyroid so far out of action that, while there is a shortage of T_4, there may be no T_3 at all, by the blood tests. In this exceptional situation it is only kind to the thyroid to help it out with tablets temporarily.

Autoimmune liver disorder quite often goes hand-in-hand with Hashimoto's type of thyroid underactivity. Obviously the latter receives treatment with thyroxine.

Kidney disorders seriously interfere with the conversion of T_4 to T_3, so that there may be less than half the usual amount of the active hormone available. This lack adds to the feelings of weakness and depression common in kidney disease. Dialysis doesn't alter the thyroid's reaction to kidney failure, but a kidney transplant restores the thyroid to normal with everything else.

Thyroid illness on top of physical illness

High blood pressure This is made worse by either an underactive or an overactive thyroid. In the former the blood vessels may get clogged with cholesterol, necessitating a higher blood pressure. In the latter the rapid heart rate raises the blood pressure directly. Either way it is vital to make sure your thyroid problem is recognized and fully treated.

Madge had always been solid, in every sense of the word. She was the backbone of the local Party HQ, the leading light in the Dramatic Society, and the driving force behind the Church-women's Guild, the Friends of the Countryside and the Summer Fete. Whatever the event, Madge was at the centre of it, organizing, commanding. At fifty she seemed unstoppable. So it was odd when Madge began missing meetings and then actually resigned from the secretaryship of the Residents' Association.

It seemed that it was all explained when the GP found she had high blood pressure. No wonder she had felt tired, said everyone. But Madge was no better after several weeks of treatment, either in her spirits or in her blood pressure. What surprised and alerted the doctor was when Madge came in muffled up in a woollen twin set on a sunny summer's day. Thyroxine for her underactive thyroid plus a beta-blocker for her blood pressure has restored Madge to her accustomed dynamic self.

Coronary heart disease Again, either clogged arteries or a pressurized heart rate, from an underactive or an overactive thyroid, adds to the risks, urgently. Treatment of the thyroid disorder has top priority.

High cholesterol (hyperlipidaemia) Underactive thyroid is the danger in this condition, which carries a possibility of stroke.

Obstructive airways problems In chronic bronchitis, emphysema and asthma the breathing problems are made worse by an overactive thyroid. You cannot take a beta-blocker to slow down the heart and breathing rates in these cases, but an antithyroid like carbimazole will make your breathing easier and more comfortable, together with your usual chest treatment.

Diabetes This illness is especially difficult to control if the thyroid is overactive, so both autoimmune disorders equally deserve full treatment.

If you have a goitre which has been no trouble over the years, if you have had a thyroid problem in the past, or if there are autoimmune disorders in the family, do not be surprised if your doctor wants to check your thyroid if you are slow to respond to treatment for any of the illnesses reviewed above. Thyroid treatment can be life-saving, or at least life-enhancing, in such cases.

Connections

Hashimoto's disease is particularly common in children and others suffering from certain genetic disorders: cystic fibrosis, Down's syndrome, Turner's syndrome, and Klinefelter's syndrome. The thyroid problem responds well to T_4 treatment in these conditions, but unfortunately does not help the genetic problem.

Graves' disorder is similarly frequently associated with ulcerative colitis, coeliac disease, Crohn's disease and myasthenia gravis.

A note for slimmers –
how to play it right

The less reputable slimming clinics often dish out 'magic pills' which contain a purgative, a diuretic, an appetite suppressant – and thyroxine. The first two cause you to lose fluid (and weight) temporarily but have no effect on fat. The thyroxine is no help either. A moderate dose will have nil effect: your own gland stops making its hormone if adequate supplies are coming in from outside. A larger dose can put a strain on the heart and cause high blood pressure, made worse in conjunction with an appetite suppressant.

Appetite suppressants all act like amphetamines, raising the blood pressure and increasing tension as inevitable side-effects. With a substantial dose of thyroxine the result can be disastrous, triggering Graves' disease, a coronary or a nervous breakdown. It is this combined effect of drugs that accounts for the deaths, from time to time, of slimmers who have fallen into the hands of the unscrupulous.

The way to get the best out of your dieting efforts and of your thyroid is by a gentler approach. If you starve yourself – or nearly – your thyroid will work against you by immediately turning your metabolic rate down, so that you use up your food and your fat at a slower rate. It will also slow down your digestion, so that you obtain every last calorie from whatever you've eaten. You will slow down generally, so that even when you exercise you will burn up fuel slowly.

It is better to reduce your weight by 1 to 2 lb weekly as a maximum, so that your thyroid is not stimulated into adjusting your metabolic rate downwards. The thyroid does not respond to your actual weight, however unacceptable to you, but to any sharp change in food intake. Since every meal you take gives your thyroid a brief boost plus an increase in metabolic rate, don't miss any meals – just change them. Cut out as far as possible the fats; don't increase the protein (meat etc.); and especially don't ditch the bread, potatoes, pasta and rice – it's carbohydrate that your thyroid runs on, and that keeps your metabolic rate up.

11

Tests and treatments

Laboratory tests are particularly useful when the thyroid is misbehaving. How you feel and what you notice wrong or unusual remain the most important aspects, but they can be deceptive. Take Graves' disease: in one person it causes a goitre, loss of weight and an anxiety state; in another, all the symptoms point to a heart disorder. A test will identify the true cause.

Reasons for having tests are:

- to check if the thyroid is working normally;
- to pinpoint the fault, if any;
- to indicate whether the problem is mild or serious;
- to help select the dosage of any medication;
- to monitor progress.

No test is 100 per cent accurate every time, but thyroid tests come close at 95 per cent.

Standard tests

These are made on a small sample of blood, and measure the concentration of various substances in it. These substances include the following:

T_4 – thyroxine, the main thyroid hormone. Each molecule contains four iodine atoms.

T_3 – triiodothyronine, the more active thyroid hormone, formed by the removal of one iodine atom from each thyroxine molecule.

rT_3 – reverse-T_3, an inactive type of T_3, with a different arrangement of its three iodine atoms.

TSH – thyroid-stimulating hormone. This is made in the pituitary gland and directs the thyroid to produce its hormones. The amount of TSH goes up when the thyroid isn't providing enough T_4 and T_3 for the body's needs, and down when there is a surplus.

TRH – thyroid-releasing hormone. This comes from the hypothalamus – the part of the brain that organizes sex, eating, drinking, sleeping and the metabolism, with an input from what's happening round you and your personal feelings and desires – and stimulates the pituitary gland to produce TSH. TRH was not discovered until 1968.

TBG – thyroid-binding globulin: one of the carrier proteins that act as transporters for 99.9 per cent of the thyroxine in the circulation.

FT_4 – free thyroxine, the tiny but significant part of this hormone in the blood which is not bound up with a protein but is immediately available. The level of this is useful for assessing whether the thyroid itself is functioning properly, regardless of the amount of carrier protein.

FT_3 – free T_3. The test for this is available in only a few laboratories.

Screening tests

Thyroid screens are used – 'just in case' – for all newborn babies in the West, for those at a key point in life, say aged sixty-five or pregnant, and for anyone with symptoms that could be caused by a thyroid problem. The usual screening tests are for T_4 or TSH.

T_4 test   This measures the amount of thyroxine in the blood, both free and attached to proteins. If the reading is below 64 international units (5 standard units), it suggests an underactive thyroid; if it is more than 142 international units (11 standard units) this should mean an overactive thyroid – other things being equal. The trouble is that other things may not be equal. If there is a shortage of carrier protein, the result will be low; an excess of protein will give a high result. Yet the thyroid may be working perfectly.

Increased protein and hence a *high* reading may be caused by:

- pregnancy, HRT or the contraceptive pill – because of the extra oestrogen;
- hepatitis – acute liver infection;
- porphyria – a rare illness affecting the skin;
- cannabis;
- just a hereditary quirk.

Reduced protein and hence a *low* reading may be caused by:

- steroids used in illness;
- body-building steroids (for athletes);
- nephrosis – a kidney problem;
- cirrhosis of the liver;
- just a hereditary quirk.

To check whether an abnormally high or low T_4 level is in fact due to the thyroid, there are two choices: the TSH or the FT_4 test.

TSH test   This is often used instead of, rather than as well as, the T_4

test; it is simpler for the lab than the FT_4 test. If the thyroid is failing to supply enough hormone for the body's requirements, TSH, the stimulator, comes into action to make the thyroid increase production. If the TSH result is above the critical level (more than 4 in either international or standard units), the thyroid simply isn't coming up with the goods: it is underactive.

If there is too much thyroxine, the thyroid needs little or no stimulation and the TSH level may be undetectable.

FT_4 test   This is becoming increasingly popular as a true measure of thyroid activity.

TBG test   This is seldom used, since thyroid function is adequately assessed without it.

T_3, FT_3 and rT_3 tests   A raised T_3 or FT_3 level occurs in T_3 toxicosis (see page 46). This causes the same symptoms as Graves' disease, but there is no excess of thyroxine, which is puzzling until the T_3 is investigated. Even with a healthy thyroid, increasing age causes a slow reduction in T_3, unlike T_4, and a number of illnesses have the same effect – the low-T_3 syndrome. Going on a fast, unwanted starvation and anorexia nervosa all induce a low T_3 level with a corresponding increase in reverse-T_3.

TRH test   Unlike those considered so far, this test involves more than taking a single blood sample. It tests the pituitary gland, which programmes the thyroid. Occasionally a low T_4 output is due to the pituitary's failing to send out the TSH to stimulate the thyroid. The test consists, essentially, of giving an injection of TRH which should stimulate a healthy pituitary to produce more TSH. The test is time-consuming but not unpleasant.

You start by missing breakfast, then have a preliminary blood test for the TSH level, and when you are lying down and mentally relaxed you are given the TRH injection. Two odd things happen: you get a funny taste in your mouth and a peculiar feeling low in your pelvic region, something like wanting to pass water. These pass off, and you have blood tests for TSH after 20, 40 and 60 minutes. Normally the TSH level increases 20 to 30 minutes after the TRH injection and goes back to its original level after 60 to 90 minutes.

If you have an overactive thyroid the TSH will not go up. It cannot if there is a pituitary disorder, nor will it in some perfectly healthy elderly men or in a serious depressive illness. The TRH test is therefore sometimes used in psychiatry to help with a diagnosis of depression, but an ordinary TSH test is simpler and just as useful to detect thyroid problems.

Antibody tests From your angle, these are simple – an ordinary blood test. For the laboratory they are complex. Antibodies in the blood indicate susceptibility to autoimmune thyroid problems:

- *Graves' disease* The main responsible antibody is TRAb – thyroid receptor antibody. If there is a high level of this during pregnancy, it is a warning to take action to protect the unborn baby.
- *Hashimoto's disease* Several antibodies are involved, including anti-Tg (antithyroglobulin)] and anti-M (antimicrosomal). 90 per cent of Hashimoto sufferers carry these antibodies, but so do 1 in 5 of people who have never had a thyroid problem. This last group may, however, be more susceptible to developing an autoimmune disorder if the thyroid is put under stress, by for instance lithium medication, an infection or a faulty diet.

Radioiodine uptake (RAIU) test This is a test of how effectively or hungrily the thyroid cells are latching on to the iodine in the circulation, which is a necessary ingredient of thyroid hormones. The test begins with a scan of your basic level of radioactivity, with a sort of Geiger counter. Then you are given a measured dose of a mildly radioactive form of iodine, ^{123}I, in a capsule or as a liquid. The thyroid area is then scanned again at various intervals up to twenty-four hours to see how much of the iodine has been taken up. For a quicker test the follow-up scan can be done three to four hours after the start, but in this case you must do without food during the whole time.

The results are useful in diagnosis and also in assessing the dosage necessary if radioiodine treatment is in view.

High uptake will result from:

- Graves' disease and other overactivity;
- iodine deficiency;
- having stopped antithyroid drugs;
- a diet full of soya;
- kidney disease.

Low uptake will result from:

- an underactive thyroid;
- medicines containing iodine;

121

- diet – 'iodine-enriched' foods or vitamin products;
- taking thyroxine – you have to stop it a month before the test;
- previous radioidine treatment or thyroid operation;
- old age;
- having just exercised very energetically.

The radioactive iodine used for the RAIU test has nothing like the strength of that used in treatment. Its radioactivity only lasts three or four days. Another radioactive material, technetium, is sometimes used instead of iodine; it is given by injection. Whichever material is used, the test is unsuitable for young children or anyone who might be pregnant, even at this low level of radiation.

Scintigram This technique uses a special camera to produce a brightly multicoloured picture showing where iodine is taken up by thyroid tissue, and how vigorously. Like the RAIU test, it depends on having a measured amount of the weak radioiodine, ^{123}I, or technetium 99m first. In a few centres fluorescent scanning is available: this measures ordinary, non-radioactive iodine through something like an X-ray, and almost no radiation is involved.

A scintigram is useful:

- to show the size and shape of the gland;
- to check for thyroid tissue behind the breastbone;
- to find out whether a lump in the tongue or neck is thyroid tissue that has gone off course during development;
- most importantly, to provide information on a particular knob or lump of tissue in the thyroid:

    – a 'hot' nodule (showing as red) is overactive, taking in a lot of iodine;
    – a 'warm' nodule (showing as orangey-yellow) is normally active;
    – a 'cold' nodule (showing as greenish) is not taking up iodine and may be a cyst or a tumour. This calls for further investigation, to exclude cancer.

X-ray An ordinary X-ray gives a shadowy idea of the size and position of the thyroid. In particular, a chest X-ray may reveal a shadow behind the breastbone which could be an extension of thyroid tissue. Ultrasound, a CT scan or a scintigram will be needed for more precise information.

Barium swallow This is an X-ray taken while you are swallowing a barium drink that shows up on X-ray. It reveals any pressure on your gullet.

CT (computerized tomography) scan   This is an X-ray that presents what looks like pictures of slices through the neck or other area.

Ultrasound   This a simple, painless method of obtaining a picture of an internal organ, including the thyroid. It is perfectly safe for pregnant mothers or children. It produces an ongoing image, a moving picture, by processing the echo of a high-frequency sound – too high for the human ear – projected on to the organ. The echoes vary depending on the consistency of the tissues under the skin. The principle is something like that of distinguishing between a piece of wood, a tin can and a cushion by tapping them. A normal thyroid is solid but not hard, but not the same as a cyst full of fluid. The technological magic is in converting the inaudible echoes into visible pictures.

The procedure is pleasant enough. You lie down and your neck is anointed with a lubricant gel or oil. The sensitive endpiece of the apparatus then slides over your skin easily, and that's all you feel.

Apart from distinguishing a cyst from solid tissue, the ultrasound provides an ongoing image of the organs and structures in your neck. This is invaluable for guiding the needle when a biopsy of a particular part of the thyroid is required.

Fine-needle aspiration (FNA)   This is a neat method of doing a biopsy – that is, obtaining a sample of tissue to examine under the microscope and identify precisely. It is safe, simple and quick. You lie down with a small pillow under your shoulders. A local anaesthetic may be used, but the aspiration is anyway almost painless. A fine needle with a syringe attached is slipped into the part to be investigated, and a tiny sample is withdrawn.

If it is a very small nodule that is to be examined, ultrasound will allow the operator to see exactly where the tip of the needle is, throughout.

The great value of FNA is for distinguishing between a common-place nodule of normal thyroid tissue, a harmless cyst or benign growth, and a cancer. This knowledge is a signpost to the best form of treatment.

Metabolic rate   Although the main work of the thyroid is control-ling the rate at which the bodily processes use up the available nourishment, the metabolic rate is seldom tested. Up till now there has been no quick and simple method, but technology is catching up. The test is useful in research studies. The principle is to assess the amount of oxygen you use, minute by minute. This goes up immediately after a meal. You may notice that you feel warmer, even after cold food, because of the increased slow combustion going on inside you.

A raised background, or basic metabolic rate goes with overactivity of the thyroid, and accounts for the person who eats enormously and stays thin. The opposite happens with an underactive thyroid.

Electrocardiogram This electrical tracing of the heart's activity is the standard method of assessing how well the heart is working. It shows characteristic changes in overactive and underactive thyroid.

Ophthalmic curve meter This apparatus measures the degree of protrusion of the eye or eyes.

Treatment for an underactive thyroid

The aim is to restore normal levels of thyroid hormone as soon as possible. If you are a young, healthy adult, and haven't been ill for more than a few months, you can start with a reasonably large dose of the synthetic thyroxine – say 100 micrograms daily, in one tiny white tablet. Usually this will need to be adjusted upwards after the first month or two. After that there will be checks of how you feel and blood tests at longer intervals.

Special circumstances Half doses for the first month are given to:

- those with years-long thyroid lack;
- those over forty-five and healthy.

Quarter doses for the first month are given to:

- those over forty and with severe thyroid lack;
- those with heart problems.

Other special cases are:

- after radioiodine treatment or surgery it takes several weeks for the remaining thyroid to settle and for the dosage of T_4 to be worked out;
- the elderly – seventy-plus – smaller doses are adequate;
- babies need full dosage (for their size) from day 1;
- children up to five years need relatively high doses.

Subclinical hypothyroidism In this state you feel perfectly well but a routine screening reveals that you have a high TSH, indicating some thyroid shortage. Your doctor may give you a trial of thyroxine or prefer just to keep an eye on your progress. This is what happened with Vivienne. A high TSH reading persisted for over a year after her last baby, but it wasn't until she was in her forties, ten years later, and had just had a bout of gastroenteritis, that the symptoms of hypothyroidism appeared.

How long to continue with the treatment Medication for an under-active thyroid is usually required for life. The dose that keeps you feeling well and your TSH level normal should be continued, with a check every six to twelve months. It may be possible to reduce it as you grow older.

Effects, good and bad Although the effects of thyroxine begin within hours of the first tablet, you will not notice any change for four or five days:

- Your pulse speeds up so your circulation is better.
- Your temperature goes up to normal, so you feel warmer.
- You pass a lot of water in the first two or three days, because your body has stored too much.
- You feel lighter because of this fluid loss, and your weight continues to go down a little as you shed the surplus fat.
- Your appearance improves – you lose the ugly puffiness, and your face is once more expressive. Gradually your skin becomes softer and smoother, and new, and the yellowish tinge disappears.
- You are livelier, more alert, happier.
- Your speech becomes faster and clearer within a week.
- Your appetite improves.
- You want to drink more, because now you are losing moisture by perspiration.
- Your bowels are freer, and your periods no longer heavy and irregular.
- Chemically, although you can't see it, the amount of cholesterol in your blood diminishes, and if you had been anaemic this also improves.

Except that it is more often a woman who is the victim, recovery from underactive thyroid is like the fairy-tale transformation of the frog into the handsome prince.

Of course taking too much thyroxine can lead to any of the

symptoms of overactive thyroid. If the dosage is built up too quickly, angina pains may crop up in those already susceptible – these are a signal to reduce the dose. Pains in other muscles arise fairly frequently in the first few weeks, but these are temporary and harmless, though unpleasant. If you are diabetic, as your metabolism speeds up with the T_4, you may need more insulin or other medication to control your sugar level. On the other hand, if you are taking digoxin for a heart condition, you may find you require less. Your doctor will advise you.

Myxoedema coma   This is a medical emergency, and there is no time to do tests before starting treatment. A huge dose of thyroxine (300 to 500 mcg) by injection or a tube to the stomach and nothing more for a week is favoured by some specialists; others prefer smaller doses of T_3 which acts quicker, or T_4 given daily. Heart, breathing and kidney functions may all need support, while hypothermia must be dealt with slowly and cautiously. It is only in hospital that the facilities are at hand.

Treatment for an overactive thyroid

Antithyroid drugs

It was during the Second World War that the first drugs for controlling thyroid overactivity were discovered – the antithyroids. They prevent the formation of thyroid hormones while you are taking them, but only in a minority do the effects continue if the medication is stopped. The three in common use are methimazole, propylthiouracil (PTU), and carbimazole. The last two also inhibit the conversion of T_4 into the more active T_3, and the formation of the antithyroid antibodies responsible for Graves' disease.

Uses   Most people with overactive thyroid who are under forty-five are given a trial of an antithyroid before any other treatment is used; a quarter of them seem to be cured. The others may need several courses to effect a permanent cure, or may remain on the medicine indefinitely, unless or until they decide to go for radioiodine therapy or an operation.

How long to continue with the treatment   Antithyroids have to be taken regularly, several times a day, particularly during the early weeks of treatment, since they do not last long in the body. This is especially important in severe cases. The dose can be increased if necessary. At best it takes four to six weeks to get the thyroid under some sort of control. By this stage, you can usually settle into a routine of taking the medicine every six to eight hours, and with PTU you may be able to remain free of symptoms on a once-daily regime.

Usually you would stay on the course for a year, but if you were only mildly affected you might like to try reducing the dose afer six months.

In over 60 per cent the symptoms creep back after three or four months, even if they've completed a twelve-month stint. Some people go the other way and gradually slip into the underactive thyroid situation – a sign of this happening is the goitre's getting bigger.

Effects, good and bad   Beneficial effects are the disappearance of anxiety, tremor, palpitations and weight loss and the other symptoms of overactive thyroid.

Unfortunately, some people are sensitive to these drugs. The commonest reactions are a slightly raised temperature and a blotchy-red, itchy rash. There may be odd pains that move from joint to joint, and swelling of the glands.

A more serious development is an interference with the production of the white blood cells – an important part of the body's defence against infection. A sore throat and feeling vaguely under par are the early warning signs of this condition, which is called agranulocytosis. They call for an urgent call to the doctor, a blood test and stopping the medication. You can then either switch to a different antithyroid or go for radioiodine treatment.

Mark was eighteen. He had been a diabetic since he was eleven, and he went to his doctor because he found that he was needing more and more insulin. The doctor noticed that he was sweating, his pulse was rapid – over 100 a minute instead of around 65 – and he had a small goitre. Tests showed an overactive thyroid, and Mark was put on PTU – propylthiouracil. This seemed to suit him: his insulin needs settled back to normal, and he felt more relaxed.

In the autumn he went away to university. He continued with the PTU but didn't bother to visit the college medic. When he saw his own doctor in the summer vacation the next year, Mark had put on more weight than he liked, looked puffy, and felt tired all the time – at nineteen! His thyroid was bigger. The medication was stopped, and a blood test showed not only a low T_4 level but a dangerous reduction in white blood cells, the body's protectors. Mark was laid-back about the whole affair, but the doctor was relieved when Mark's blood count started improving within days of withholding the antithyroid. After a month his goitre had shrunk to half its size, and he became his usual lively self.

Now he is nearing the end of his course and the whole thyroid saga is history. He is on no medication for his thyroid, and shows no signs of lack of hormone or too much. Nevertheless, it is clear that this young man will be susceptible to autoimmune disorders all his life – especially when he is under some physical or mental strain. It was probably partly because of A levels and girlfriend problems that he slipped into thyroid overactivity that first summer. And there is a particularly close association between Mark's autoimmune type of diabetes (insulin-dependent) and both Graves' and Hashimoto's thyroid disorders.

Apart from their use as a control and a possible cure for overactive thyroid, antithyroids are frequently used short-term, in the run-up to radioiodine or surgical treatment. The side-effects are less likely to cause trouble during so limited a period.

Beta-blockers

These modern drugs are in common use – for angina, high blood pressure, anxiety states, tremor, overactive thyroid, and sometimes migraine. What they block are the stimulating nerve pathways of the autonomic nervous system – the network which controls the heartbeat and other bodily functions we take for granted. The first and standard beta-blocker is propranolol; others are nadolol, atenolol and metoprolol (their names all end in 'olol'). They have no direct effect on the thyroid, except to inhibit mildly the conversion of T_4 to T_3, but they are useful in overactive thyroid for their other actions.

Because they act quickly, they are helpful in the early stages of treatment in Graves' disease, before the antithyroid has taken effect, but they are not suitable for prolonged use, or as the only treatment, since they have no curative value. They are often useful during the preparation period before radioiodine or surgical treatment, when the overactivity of the gland must be quietened down. People who are sensitive to antithyroids rely on beta-blockers for this.

How to take them Beta-blockers come as capsules or tablets. Some preparations have to be taken several times a day, but, once you have established what dosage suits you, there are slow-release formulations which you need take only once a day.

Precautions   You must not take beta-blockers if you are asthmatic or have ever had obstructive airways disease or heart block. They are not suitable if you are breast-feeding or in the last weeks of pregnancy, and they tend to make diabetes slightly worse. Some medicines do not mix well with beta-blockers, so remind your doctor if you are on any of these: amiodarone, tranquillizers, sleepers, antidiabetic drugs, and water tablets – and go easy on alcohol.

Effects, good and bad   On the plus side are a restful slowing of your heart rate, calming down of palpitations or tremor, and keeping you cool physically and emotionally. The side-effects, which affect only a minority, include tummy disturbance, feeling drained, difficulty with erections, bad dreams, and very rarely a rash or dry eyes. These unpleasant symptoms improve as soon as you stop taking the medicine.

Iodine and iodide

These are given in a capsule or more often as drops of Lugol's solution in milk or water, three times a day. Each is used as the final tuning-up before either a thyroid operation for overactive thyroid or radioiodine. You won't be taking it for more than ten days maximum.

Effects   Each rapidly cuts the production of thyroid hormones, but loses its effect within a few weeks. People who are sensitive to it may react with a runny nose, headache, sore eyes or a rash. It is not suitable for anyone pregnant or breast-feeding, and would thoroughly upset the thyroid if you stayed on it too long.

Radioiodine

Radioiodine (^{131}I) has revolutionized thyroid treatment, replacing the disappointing antithyroid drugs, which nearly always fail in the end, and making unnecessary in most cases the difficult operation for removing part or all of the gland. One dose of radioiodine, or at most two or three, is all that is needed to tame the most unruly overactive thyroid. You don't even need to stay in hospital overnight.

129

Who can prescribe it? Only a doctor with a licence to do so, based on special knowledge and experience.

Precautions You cannot have this treatment if you are pregnant or breast-feeding. In fact if you are a woman in the reproductive age range it is safest to have a pregnancy test first, and then have the treatment in the first ten days of your monthly cycle. Nor should you be planning a pregnancy for another six months. Apart from these circumstances, no age or sex is a barrier, and, specifically, radioiodine can be given safely to growing children.

Who should take it? This is the treatment *par excellence* for Graves' disease or toxic multinodular or single-nodule goitre. It is also used in thyroid cancers as a fail-safe follow-on to surgery. It doesn't help in de Quervain's thyroiditis (see page 24), and in Graves' disease with severe eye problems it is just possible it could make them worse.

Preliminaries To guard against the dangerous reaction of 'thyroid storm', a major upset of the gland in reaction to the sudden change in thyroid hormone production (see page 63), if you have even a moderately severely overactive thyroid you must take the edge off the disorder before you have the radioiodine. During two to eight weeks before the day, you must have a course of one of the antithyroid drugs, such as carbimazole. This stops three or four days before you are due to have the radioiodine, to ensure that the thyroid will take in as much of the medicine as possible. Some doctors may also give you propranolol, and in the last ten days, before four-day stopping of the thyroid-calming drugs, some iodine drops.

The dosage of radioiodine will be worked out in advance according to your size and the severity of your symptoms. This may be assisted by a radioiodine uptake (RAIU) test, which would have to be done before the antithyroid was started (see page 121).

Taking radioiodine It couldn't be simpler: you swallow it in a drink or as capsules and go home the same day. You remain slightly radioactive to other people for a few days, and have to take a few simple precautions for their sake – see page 50 for details.

Effects, good and bad The benefits aren't instant, but there is a 50 to 75 per cent chance of having a normally working thyroid gland within two months, and the goitre will have become visibly smaller.

If the overactivity symptoms – weight loss, palpitations, anxiety, fast pulse, loose motions etc. – are still with you, it is easy to have another dose of the medicine. The chances of a relapse are almost nil, compared with 10 per cent after an operation and 60 per cent of those on antithyroids.

You may get a feeling of warmth or discomfort in your neck temporarily after radioiodine, and occasionally the sudden change from too much T_4 to too little may bring on aching and stiffness in your muscles and joints. This is quickly cured by a short course of thyroxine tablets. The most likely unwanted effect of the radio-iodine treatment is the development of underactivity of the thyroid. The slow-down symptoms may appear after a few months and recover without help over another few weeks, or they may develop over some years and remain permanently (see below).

Some people notice a thinning of their hair two to three months after radioiodine. This is more a part of the recovery process than a side-effect. It is temporary and requires no treatment.

Follow-up treatment Sometimes there is a blip of increased excess-thyroid symptoms immediately after the radioiodine, but in any case the original symptoms will reappear. They are likely to take some weeks to subside, as the radioactivity bites. You can take a beta-blocker right away to tide you over this period, and after a couple of weeks you can take an antithyroid again, until it is no longer necessary.

If the thyroid reacts by switching down almost at once into underactivity after the radioiodine, it is not usually worthwhile to take thyroxine for what may be a short-lived fall-off in hormone production. If you have persistently low thyroxine and symptoms, then you cetainly need to start taking the tablets – probably for life. Fortunately they are so little trouble.

Surgical treatment

Surgical removal of part of the thyroid gland, under a general anaesthetic, cuts down on overproduction of the hormones and is an effective cure for Graves' disease and the other types of over-activity. It is the obvious choice if antithyroid drugs have failed or cause side-effects and radioiodine is ruled out. The latter may be because of a pregnancy planned or under way, breast-feeding, strong feelings against radioactive treatment, or work or study commitments that make impractical the prolonged medical follow-up necessary with radioiodine. Anyone with severe eye symptoms may not care to risk the possibility of radioiodine making them worse. Other reasons to choose surgery are a large, unsightly or awkwardly situated goitre or a suspicion of cancer.

Surgery is not advisable for anyone with serious heart or chest problems, or in the last three months of pregnancy.

Preliminaries To cut the risk of 'thyroid storm' (see page 63), much the same precautions are needed as before radioiodine treatment. An antithyroid is given for some weeks – as long as it takes to settle the thyroid to near-normality – and, in the last week or ten days before the operation, iodine drops are added. With surgery there is no need to stop these medicines days before the operation.

Effects, good and bad Surgery is the quickest way to be rid of the symptoms of overactive thyroid permanently. Nowadays it is an extremely safe operation, but there are possible complications.

- *Speech* The nerves to the vocal cords run across the thyroid, and may be bruised, irritated or even cut during surgery. The effect is a husky voice, which usually recovers over a few months. Repair of a seriously damaged nerve may be made up to two to three months later.
- *Low calcium in the blood (hypocalcaemia)* In a small minority the calcium-controlling parathyroid glands are damaged by thyroid surgery (see page 103). The symptoms are numbness round the mouth, tingling and muscle cramps. Calcium tablets, or an injection, put matters right. Long-term lack of parathyroid hormone can occur and calls for different management (see page 103).
- *Underactive thyroid* Some people, though not as many as with radioiodine treatment, gradually slip into this state and will require indefinite hormone replacement in the form of thyroxine.

Treatment of thyroid cancer

An operation to remove the tumour and surrounding tissue is the first step, and no preliminary antithyroid treatment is needed. High doses of radioiodine – double those used for treating Graves' disease – are given to nullify any remaining harmful thyroid cells. If there is some reason preventing an operation, for instance a bad heart, radioiodine treatment alone is effective. It is also useful for locating and dealing with any secondary tumours that might appear.

Effects, good and bad In most types of thyroid cancer, the cancerous tissue and some natural thyroid is removed or put out of action. The success rate tops 90 per cent. The unwanted effects include temporary swelling and discomfort in the neck, and sometimes a brief surge of thyroid hormone into the bloodstream speeds up the heart and causes anxiety feelings. This settles within days. The other unwanted reactions soon after treatment are the headache and muscle and joint problems mentioned in the treatment of overactive thyroid (page 127). They are a reminder to start on thyroxine tablets, which will deal with the symptoms and which you are bound to require for the future.

Treatment of goitre

The first essential is a T_4 or TSH test to find out whether the thyroid is underactive or overactive.

Smooth, symmetrical enlargement

If the thyroid is underactive, the treatment is thyroxine tablets. If overactive, antithyroid or radioiodine treatment. If the gland is functioning normally you can ignore the situation or you may opt for a six-month trial of T_4 to see if this will induce the goitre to shrink. Keep alert for any symptoms of too much thyroid – palpitations, anxiety and tremor.

If the goitre is very large, uncomfortable or ugly, and it won't shrink with medical treatment, surgery is the only option.

Irregular, knobbly goitre

If the goitre is small, it may shrink sufficiently with thyroxine in the case of an underactive or normal gland, or with antithyroid or radioiodine if it is overactive. Probably these treatments won't change the size and look of the goitre, so if it is troubling you at all you should get it removed by surgery and take T_4 hormone replacement if necessary.

Single nodule

This is nearly always safest and best removed, since you can never be sure whether it might become cancerous. It would not require a big operation, since only the nodule need go.

Endemic and iodine-deficiency goitres

Millions of people in Asia and Africa have these goitres, and in some districts they are accepted as normal. They can become enormous, but the worst aspect is that many are associated with a devastating deficiency of thyroid hormones. Children are stunted and mentally impaired, and the adults are dull and squat.

Effective treatment must be preventive, and usually consists of the large-scale distribution of salt, bread or some other staple which has been iodized, plus a cleaning-up of water supplies. Highly successful programmes have been run in Switzerland, Mexico and Argentina.

Iodized oil by injection, lasting three years, or by mouth, lasting three months, is useful in the preventive treatment of pregnant women and young children who live in the less sophisticated parts of the world.

Treatment of eye problems

Eye problems arise mainly in Graves' disease, but occasionally in Hashimoto's. Either way they are due to a special autoimmune process. Smoking has been proven to make eye problems likelier, or worse if they are present. Cutting out smoking is a must.

Mild cases need only mild treatment, while the thyroid disorder itself is being brought under control. Dark glasses with flaps on the sides to protect your eyes from irritating gusts of wind and dust are helpful. Demulcent eyedrops, usually hypromellose, put in every two to three hours, keep the surface of the eye lubricated and soothed. Racing goggles such as swimmers use look weird but may help, and it may be more comfortable for your eyes if you sleep with the head of the bed raised up a few inches. Some people find the swelling is reduced if they take water tablets. In any event, in mild cases the outlook is excellent.

Severe cases There are several lines of treatment. Steroids are usually given to reduce the swelling, in a course that tapers off over two months, but if you are over fifty you may not be able to take full doses of steroids because of side-effects like raised blood pressure. Radiation therapy is effective in more than half of those for whom other treatment has failed, and some physicians make radiation their first choice. Surgery allows more room for the swollen eyes, but a second operation is often necessary to get the eye muscles in balance. Of course, improvement in the thyroid overactivity is important, but unfortunately it is not the whole answer.

General treatment of thyroid sufferers

Although the specific treatments are vital, so also is comprehensive physical and psychological care. All the disorders that affect the thyroid are both physically and emotionally upsetting in a variety of ways. While you are struggling to recover in the early days of treatment, whether by tablets or by something more dramatic, indulge in a convalescent lifestyle.

For a start you need adequate rest, in non-stressful surroundings. Perhaps your body has been under strain, trying to do all the usual things without enough thyroid hormone for any part to run properly. On the other hand, with an overactive thyroid it may have been functioning at breakneck speed, to exhaustion point.

To balance up regular sleep at night, some of the daytime must be spent in exercise – the sort you do indoors to limber up, and walking or any sport you enjoy in the fresh air. Your diet must be sufficiently mixed to include all the vitamins and minerals naturally (see Chapter 10), with plenty of fruit, vegetables and protein. Fats are not particularly useful, and they are definitely out if your thyroid has not been making enough hormone. In general, if your thyroid is recovering from overactivity, you should eat more than most people while you build up what you have lost. If your thyroid was underactive you don't need to alter your food intake: the increase in metabolic rate from the extra thyroxine will be enough to level out your weight.

The strain on your emotional system will tend you towards depression with too little thyroid, or anxiety with too much. Either way, strands of both moods will be mixed together. Whichever way your thyroid has played up, your concentration, attention span and short-term memory will be substandard. You could easily lose your temper or burst into tears, and you won't have your usual efficiency. This is real suffering, and the treatment calls for a temporary lifting of day-to-day responsibilities plus lashings of sympathy, support and encouragement. It is not a for-ever situation, and you will get back to normal all the sooner if at this stage you don't struggle to take on every task or to make every decision.

If anyone offers to spoil you for a brief period, accept it. If no one else does, spoil yourself. Consider your comfort and pleasure first, postpone dealing with problems or making major plans, and concentrate on gentle diversions. Spend time with people who make you feel relaxed. You didn't choose to be ill, so cash in on the bonus side for a limited period only – say two to three weeks.

Index